Combining Psychotherapy and Drug Therapy in Clinical Practice

Combining Psychotherapy and Drug Therapy in Clinical Practice

Edited by

Bernard D. Beitman, M.D.
Department of Psychiatry and Behavioral Sciences
University of Washington School of Medicine
Seattle, Washington

Gerald L. Klerman, M.D.
Department of Psychiatry
Harvard Medical School
Massachusetts General Hospital
Boston, Massachusetts

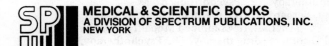

MEDICAL & SCIENTIFIC BOOKS
A DIVISION OF SPECTRUM PUBLICATIONS, INC.
NEW YORK

SPECTRUM PUBLICATIONS, INC.
175-20 Wexford Terrace
Jamaica, NY 11432

Library of Congress Cataloging in Publication Data
Main entry under title:

Combining psychotherapy and drug therapy in clinical
   practice.

   Includes bibliographies and index.
   1. Psychotherapy.   2. Psychotropic drugs.
I. Beitman, Bernard D.   II. Klerman, Gerald L.,
1928-   . [DNLM: 1. Combined Modality Therapy.
2. Mental Disorders—drug therapy.   3. Psychotherapy.
WM 402 C731]
RC480.5.C577   1984   616.89′1   84-14144
ISBN 0-89335-214-4

Printed in the United States of America

Epigraph

Increasing conscious control of one's own brain biochemistry is a major goal of research in clinical psychiatry.

Contributors

Bernard D. Beitman, M.D.   Assistant Professor, Department of Psychiatry and Behavioral Sciences, University of Washington School of Medicine, Seattle, Washington

Charles W. Bodemer, Ph.D.   Professor, Department of Biomedical History, University of Washington School of Medicine, Seattle, Washington

Albert S. Carlin, Ph.D.   Associate Professor, Department of Psychiatry and Behavioral Sciences, University of Washington School of Medicine, Seattle, Washington

John A. Chiles, M.D.   Associate Professor, Department of Psychiatry and Behavioral Sciences, University of Washington School of Medicine, Seattle, Washington

Elke D. Eckert, M.D.   Associate Professor, Department of Psychiatry, University of Minnesota, Minneapolis, Minnesota

Michael J. Goldstein, Ph.D.   Professor, Department of Psychology, University of California at Los Angeles, Los Angeles, California

Katherine A. Halmi, M.D.   Professor, Department of Psychiatry, Cornell Medical School, Ithaca, New York

Gerald L. Klerman, M.D.   Professor, Department of Psychiatry, Harvard Medical School, Boston, Massachusetts

Matig R. Mavissakalian, M.D.   Associate Professor of Psychiatry, University of Pittsburgh, Pittsburgh, Pennsylvania; Western Psychiatric Institute-Clinic, Pittsburgh, Pennsylvania

A. John Rush, M.D.   Professor, Department of Psychiatry, Southwestern Medical School, Dallas, Texas

Nicholas G. Ward, M.D.   Associate Professor, Department of Psychiatry and Behavioral Sciences, University of Washington School of Medicine, Seattle, Washington

Myrna M. Weissman, Ph.D.   Professor, Depression Research Unit, Department of Psychiatry, Yale University School of Medicine, New Haven, Connecticut

Preface

The appearance of this volume is timely and relevant. Over the past decades, there has been wide application of pharmacotherapy in the treatment of psychiatric disorders. The combination of pharmacotherapy and psychotherapy is increasingly being utilized not only by psychiatrists, but by psychologists, social workers, and other non-medical mental health professionals. Although this practice has grown, relatively little attention has been paid to its theoretical basis, scientific evidence, and clinical application in the literature and in teaching efforts.

The early 1950s witnessed the introduction of chlorpromazine, the first modern psychopharmacologic agent based upon the research of Delay and Deniker in France. The first use of chlorpromazine in North America was reported by Lehmann in 1954. Soon afterwards, a number of other classes of compounds with proven efficacy were developed, particularly the tricyclic antidepressants, the monoamine oxidase inhibitors, and the minor tranquilizers, first meprobamate and recently the benzodiazapine series.

At first, the claims for the efficacy of these compounds were met with skepticism, particularly by psychotherapists and others committed to a psychological or environmental approach to mental illness. Nevertheless, the large number of well-controlled randomized trials soon demonstrated the efficacy of these compounds over and above placebo. The question then arose as to how these new treatments compared with psychotherapy and whether there might be any benefit from combined therapy. The early efforts in this area were with schizophrenic patients. Most notable was the study by May and associates in California, which compared drugs with psychotherapy and the combination of both and demonstrated that drug therapy was more effective than psychotherapy alone, but there was some advantage to the combination.

The research literature grew; initial studies of schizophrenia were extended to studies in depression, agoraphobia, anorexia nervosa and obesity. Clinical practice has often been ahead of research efforts on purely pragmatic grounds. Clinicians, particularly those not bound by adherence to ideological positions, began to explore various combinations of drugs and psychotherapy. These efforts took place in inpatient settings, in outpatient clinics, and in the offices of individual practitioners.

The current scene is one in which there is widespread acceptance among clinicians of the value of combined therapy. Recent surveys in the State of Washington, reported in this volume by Chiles et al, indicate that the majority of psychiatrists and psychologists are actively involved in combined therapy and that various arrangements for interprofessional collaboration and cooperation have evolved. New forms of psychotherapeutic practice have had to be developed to enhance the psychological management of patients receiving drug therapy and to respond to the interpersonal complexities of the psychotherapy-pharmacotherapy triangle in which pharmacotherapy is administered by an MD, usually a psychiatrist, and psychotherapy is administered by a nonphysician, usually a psychologist or social worker. These new areas of clinical practice are rapidly changing; the work reported in this volume by Beitman, Ward, and Chiles summarize the current state of knowledge and experience and contribute to improving clinical practice.

At the same time that clinical practice has evolved, the quality of research projects has extended greatly as reflected in the chapters in Part 3. Individual reports on combined treatment for depression, schizophrenia, agoraphobia, and anorexia nervosa test the growing sophistication in the research community and reveal the complexity of findings with theoretical and clinical relevance. It is likely that this volume will be the first of a series. As clinical experience and the range of clinical application of combined treatment extends, future reports will summarize these new developments.

Gerald L. Klerman
Bernard D. Beitman

Contents

III. SPECIFIC DIAGNOSTIC CATEGORIES

Acknowledgments

Jack Lein, M.D., saw enough promise in a modest proposal for a Continuing Medical Education Program at the University of Washington to vault it into the first national symposium on clinical combined therapy. At the last moment, representatives of Ciba–Geigy and Mead Johnson provided travel funds for speakers at the August 4–6, 1983, meeting who might not otherwise have been able to attend. Pat Lind, of the Continuing Medical Education Program, shepherded the details into a successful final outcome. Linda Crew, with back-up assistance from Lorraine Fitz, provided the quickly responsive administrative and secretarial help to make the conference and this book a reality. Jane Borstel was supportive and determined at times when all looked bleak. And Paula Levine helped to sharpen the presentation of Chapters 3 and 4 with her clear copyediting.

History and Ideology

CHAPTER 1

Historical Perspectives on Combined Treatment

Charles W. Bodemer

This presentation examines the background to the evolution of combined therapy within the context of the history of psychiatry. A distinctive feature of that history is the powerful conditioning effect of the intellectual and cultural environment. Thus, because of prevailing philosophical and religious perceptions of human nature and the orientation of Western civilization, psychiatry as such did not develop until the late 18th century. The medieval period was critical to this development, for then the writing of Augustine and Aquinas combined with the dogma and activities of the Church to determine the content of psychological theory, explanations of psychopathology, and the role of the physician in treatment of the mentally ill.

THE MEDIEVAL LEGACY

Augustine emerges as the outstanding psychologist of Western antiquity. His autobiographical *Confessions* is a remarkable psychological treatise, the earliest in Western civilization to deal with developmental psychology, motivation, social determinants of behavior, and memory [1]. Augustine's demonstration that introspection is an important source of genuine psychological knowledge was a significant contribution to psychology and locates him as a fifth century forerunner of phenomenology and psychoanalysis. Like other Patristic writers, Augustine was preoccupied with the soul, and when he equated the theological soul with the rational principle in man, he determined the future orientation of psychological thought and psychological medicine.

Augustine created the foundation for the Scholastic interpretation of human nature and psychology formulated by Thomas Aquinas during the 13th century [2]. Like Augustine, Aquinas considered the soul to be incorporeal and immortal; like Aristotle, he stressed the utility of body and soul into a compound entity. He was, however, a dualist and argued that the unified body-soul compound is inextricably linked with bodily functions, including the senses and memory, whereas the spiritual soul is responsible only for acts of reasoning and volition. Reason or mind is thus conceived to be quite independent of the body.

Aquinas was the most influential of medieval students of psychology, and his views dominated subsequent thought. Thomistic preternaturalism was therefore important in determining medieval and early modern attitudes. Aquinas recognized the existence of extraordinary forces verging on the supernatural. Preternatural beliefs in the reality of spirits, demons, possession, and miraculous cures were widely accepted by the 13th century; Aquinas gave them new form and vigor. Preternatural phenomena, he argued, are relatively rare, unpredictable, and due to a superior power which is either benevolent when attributed to a good spirit or malevolent when attributed to an evil spirit or demon. This Scholastic benediction of preternaturalism and the concept of demoniacal possesion as a basis for psychopathology had great portent for medicine.

The Thomistic view of suffering had medical significance also. Aquinas considered the suffering of sinners to be divinely ordained, a consequence of the demands of justice immanent in the ordered universe which require the punishment of sinners. Thus, God is the author of the penalty. The pangs of conscience are a major cause of suffering and belong to the wages of sin. The guilt-laden sinner may appeal to God and religious leaders for absolution or atonement and relief of suffering. Similarly, the individual afflicted with what St. John of the Cross called "the dark night of the soul" must turn to God with a certain heedfulness and undergo a supernatural process of purification and relief of suffering. The Church, then, is the source of care and comfort, psychotherapy a function of priests.

Consolidation of the view that psychological disorders are disorders of the soul resulting from sin or preternatural causes and to be treated by religious authority resulted in the separation of psychological matters from the province of medicine. This sunderance was especially destructive after the rise of Satanism and belief in witchcraft late in the medieval period. Medical psychology then was permeated with abstract theological concepts, mental disease was attributed to sin, and sex was considered to be the major sin of mankind and the primary preoccupation of the Devil. Devils, *incubi* and *succubi*, were presumed to engage in the perennial seduction of men and women, and phenomena ranging from crop failure to male impotence were considered the handiwork of Satan and his allies. The Devil and witches clearly threatened the moral and social order. After 1484, witchcraft was defined as heresy, and authorities vigorously pursued those allied with the Author of Evil [3]. Because the psychologically impaired were usually considered victims or servants of Satan, they suffered inordinately throughout the centuries-long witchcraft craze, and those few physicians who spoke in their behalf [4] were advised to limit their attentions to organic disorders. The physician was of no consequence in the problems of salvation, preservation of the faith, suppression of sedition, and destruction of Satan's minions.

PHILOSOPHY AND PSYCHIATRY
IN THE EARLY MODERN PERIOD

Medical psychology was in a state of total arrest as the cultural movement known as the Renaissance emerged within the fabric of the waning Middle Ages. The period marks the beginning of a new interest in the study of man, including his mental processes. For the first time since antiquity, major philosophers studied psychology in isolation from theology; during the 17th century there appeared masterly works of psychological content that initiated two major themes in psychology with eventual impact upon medicine.

Perhaps the only novelty in the works of Descartes is the errors; but, nonetheless, they exerted powerful influence in the history of psychiatry by establishing a dualism underlying the modern "mind-body" problem. In his search for epistemologic certainty [5], Descartes adopted an attitude of absolute scepticism leading him to conclude that "my essence consists solely in the fact that I am a thinking thing," and that "the soul by which I am what I am is entirely and absolutely distinct from my body." Descartes viewed animals as automata governed by strict laws of physics, and in his nonbiological orientation, mind became virtually independent of organic matrix. The brain was required for imagination and sensation, but cognition or "pure intelligence" was an inextended substance, *sui generis* and independent of physical laws. Except for the bridge provided by the pineal gland, the independence of mind and body was complete. Cartesian mechanism and dualism adumbrated a psychology divorced from physics and physiology. When occasionalists like Malebranche eliminated even the pineal bridge, the resulting parallelism, positing that mind and body act harmoniously but independently, rendered it reasonable to advocate study of one without reference to the other. By implication, psychology belonged to one world, physics to another.

The nature of *res cogitans* and the concept of innate ideas constituted a challenge to the ardent empiricist Locke. Locke denied the Cartesian concept of human understanding as an innate predisposition according with inherent categories of understanding [6]. Repudiating the notion of innate ideas, he made sensory experience the foundation of knowledge. Condillac later espoused his version of the Lockean view in France [7], where it profoundly affected the course of psychiatry.

During the Age of Reason, mental illness began to escape the fetters of superstition and authoritarian error. The physiological orientation of physicians and the stunted state of psychological medicine precluded any rapid developments, but there were clear indications of change. Linnaean codification was ascendant in the natural sciences, and psychiatric nosology occupied the attention of many 18th century physicians [8]. The psychiatric taxonomists did not advance understanding of psychological miseries, nor did they seriously affect the existing methods of treatment. Boerhaave's psychotherapy, for example, continued to consist of bloodletting and purgatives, ice-water baths, and a form of shock-treatment wherein a spinning chair rendered the patient unconcious. Significantly, however, during this period physicians began to study and treat psychiatric disabilities; the care and comfort of the mentally ill was no longer an activity properly claimed by ecclesiastical authority alone.

The Enlightenment is a turning point in the history of psychiatry. The treatment of the mentally ill was revolutionized, especially by Pinel, who installed a therapeutic program embodying sensationalist psychology and Enlightenment ideals at the institutions under his direction [9]. Pinel's "moral treatment" was a form of restraint-free therapy based on the Lockean assumption that sensory impressions underlie neural function and that ideas and emotions relate to external stimuli. Moral treatment depended upon regulation of the environment so as to reduce the psychologically disturbing stimuli, calm the passions or emotions, and restore the disturbed person's rational faculties and normal behavior. The medical model of psychopathology originated during the Enlightenment. Pinel expressed it well: "The mentally ill, far from being guilty persons who merit punishment, are sick people whose miserable state deserves all the consideration due to suffering humanity." Moreover, psychiatry as a medical discipline dates from the time Pinel employed physicians to care for the patients at Bicêtre and Salpêtrière. Psychiatry thus originated in institutions and was represented for decades by the medical superintendents of the 19th century asyla.

THE 19th CENTURY REIGN OF SOMATICISM

Nineteenth century medicine shed metaphysics and adopted physicochemical methods and techniques in the attempt to become a natural science. Analysis of the nervous system progressed steadily, and most investigations revealed a relation of localized structure and function. This encouraged growth of somato-pathological approaches in psychological medicine and a corresponding tendency to disparage psychological approaches. By the 1870s, most practitioners assumed the superior efficacy and scientific validity of the somatic approach and agitated for a reclassification of mental disorders on systematic and somato-pathological principles conforming with knowledge of cerebral localization. The psychological approach to behavioral problems was emphatically rejected, and the psychological interpretation of symptoms was utilized only for diagnostic purposes.

Treatment of psychiatric diseases consisted almost entirely in the treatment of concurrent bodily disease through medicinal and regimenal means.

The exclusion of psychological and psychotherapeutic approaches from 19th century psychiatry derived primarily from the thoroughly dualistic interpretation of mental illness [10,11]. The body was believed to comprise separate psychological and physiological systems, whose processes were relatively autonomous and governed by different principles. These systems coexisted in a certain equilibrium, but they normally didn't interact or influence each other directly. Normal mentation and voluntary behavior were self-determined, albeit subject to the uniform and universal "laws of mind" given by association psychology. Normal vital processes were firmly determined and governed in a separate sphere by the "laws of organization" given by the biological and physical sciences. Normal physiological processes underlay vital phenomena accomplished without the intervention or arousal of consciousness. States of consciousness were the result of normal psychological processes, subject to the Will and its power determinately to focus the individual's attention on particular sensations, ideas, and motivations. Such healthy minds perceived external reality correctly, formed correspondingly intelligent judgments, and allowed for appropriate conduct. Mental health was the degree to which those powers were retained that served to sustain the control of the Will and the associated powers of reason. Mental illness was considered to result from the reduction or loss of the natural autonomy of psychological processes. Removed from volitional control and deprived of self-determination, thought and feeling were reduced either to epiphenomena of underlying morbid structural or functional states of the brain especially or they were eliminated altogether. Behavior degenerated *pari passu*, becoming more reflex, implusive, and irresponsible in character. The differential view of mind-body relations thus led to the identification of mental illness as the loss of the natural autonomy of the psychic life and its domination by the physical. This assumed etiology led naturally to medical, rather than psychotherapeutic, treatment.

Clinical, as opposed to institutional, psychiatry developed as a part of 19th century neurology [12-15]. Neurologic and psychiatric diseases alike received physiological explanations, and insanity was viewed as a symptom-complex of abnormal states of the brain. Establishment of the somato-pathological stance and the almost universal interpretation of insanity as a result of structural or functional lesions of the "organ of mind" entrenched the medical model of psychopathology; medicine appropriated and cultivated mental disorders as a rightful sphere of professional involvement. The cleric dealing with disorders of the soul yielded to the neuropsychiatrist dealing with disorders of the brain, and at century's end Kraepelin's *Lehrbuch* rose as a monument defining psychiatry as a medical discipline theoretically free of poetic and moralistic attitudes [16].

Nineteenth century medicine strove to acquire the rationality and epistemological rigor developed in the physical sciences; forms of explanation divergent from received ideas of scientific naturalism were suspect. The implications of this attitude became manifest in the restriction of legitimate medical psychology to the sphere of diagnosis and an insistence upon established physiological rationales to legitimate the medical use of psychological methods of treatment [17,18]. The prevailing medical concept of psychopathology, however, effectively frustrated development of such rationales. As long as the brain was considered to comprise the organ of mind conditioning all its manifestations, the mind itself couldn't be diseased and medical treatment necessarily had to focus upon its organ. Attempts to operate directly upon the mind could not win acceptance in the absence of a convincing physiological rationale for whatever degree of efficacy they appeared to possess. Anything less was unscientific and therefore unacceptable. The fervent pursuit of the scientific habitus clarifies the development within orthodox medicine of a general and inflexible hostility toward psychological methods of treatment. This hostility underlay the splenetic disdain for available evidence concerning psychosomatic phenomena and the rejection of mesmerism and hypnotism as therapeutic techniques.

THE MODERN ORIGINS OF PSYCHOTHERAPY

During the late 18th century, Mesmer obtained extraordinarily successful therapeutic results with a method he called "animal magnetism" [19]. Mesmer believed that man's health depended upon the amount and distribution of a universal magnetic fluid within the body. Cures were obtained through physical contact with a magnetist or objects charged with magnetic power. Rebuffed by a Royal Commission, Mesmer retired from public life, but mesmerism didn't depart with its creator. It was cultivated especially by

Puységur, who published observations on "artificial somnambulism," a sleep-like state that often occurred during mesmeric treatment [20]. Some in the early 19th century realized that psychological forces were operative in this somnambulism and that it didn't require contact with magnetist or objects. This idea didn't become widespread, however, until around mid-century and publication of Braid's treatise introducing the terms hypnosis and suggestion [21]. Braid provided a physiological explanation for mesmeric phenomena, but the conditioning intellectual environment severely blunted the possible impact of his work. The increasing association of mesmerism with phrenology and the atmosphere of deliberate mystification, quackery, and dubious morality surrounding it engendered an attitude within the medical profession that compounded the general hostility toward psychotherapy. Orthodox medical psychology therefore dismissed Braid's argument that mesmeric manipulation and hypnotism be admitted to the therapeutic armamentarium on an experimental basis and evaluated independently of the theory of animal magnetism.

It is paradoxical that neurology, the citadel of somaticism, produced the pioneers in psychogenic research. Nineteenth century neurologists, however, were practicing official psychiatry of neuroses and faced an apparent epidemic of neurasthenia, a wondrous mélange of complaints since described as neurotic, functional, or psychosomatic [22]. Similarly, hysteria was a functional neurosis frequently encountered in neurological practice. Hysteria claimed the attention of Charcot with results affecting the future development of psychotherapy. Studying it as he studied other nervous diseases (after 1878 using hypnosis), he concluded that hysteria was a disease of the internal capsule and hypnosis a pathological state [23]. Charcot's influence on the development of psychiatry was in the performance, not the results, of his work. He misunderstood hysteria, but his work encouraged its study; his interpretation of hypnosis was erroneous, but he made it a legitimate field of investigation and treatment. The results were new facts, new theories, undoubted therapeutic successes, and the emergence of modern psychotherapy.

The modern approach to psychotherapy originated primarily from Liébault and Bernheim at Nancy. The former concluded that suggestion was the main factor in mesmeric treatment, but his treatise of 1866 [24] joined that of Braid in the realm of the ignored. In the 1880s, Bernheim championed Liébault's methods, attained good results from their practical application, and triumphed in a controversy with the Charcot school. Bernheim argued that suggestion was essential to successful treatment with hypnosis and provided the long-sought physiological rationale for the psychotherapeutic approach [25]. A golden age of hypnosis followed, and, although a negative reaction developed at century's end, the hostility toward psychological methods in medicine waned and conditions favored their incorporation into psychiatric practice.

Psychotherapeutic and psychogenic ideas were abroad during the 1880s, a crucial decade in the history of psychiatry. It was not coincidental that Janet and Tuke in 1884 and Charcot, Déjerine, and Freud in 1886 worked with so psychogenic a subject as male hysteria. The phenomenon reflected changing medical attitudes, growing disenchantment with extreme somaticism in neuropsychiatry, and the cultural environment of *fin de siècle* Europe. Neurologists pioneered because, unlike the psychiatrists, who saw only institutionalized psychotics, they dealt with patients who could profit from psychotherapeutic techniques. Therapeutic successes did not necessarily imply genuine knowledge of etiology or causal treatment; however, the fact that many neurotic and some psychotic patients actually improved as a result of psychotherapy was a substantial achievement for the time and accounts for its final acceptance within medicine. The speculative aspects and other weaknesses of the early psychogenic movement may be criticized, but it should be remarked that somaticists like Meynert indulged in speculation, and the religious character sometimes assumed by psychoanalysis was not absent in scientific movements like Darwinism. Importantly, it liberated psychiatry from a spirit of hopelessness and sterility and represented an advance beyond observation of the external manifestations of total disease processes to an appreciation and limited understanding of the processes themselves.

TWENTIETH CENTURY TRENDS AND DEVELOPMENTS

Throughout the 20th century there have been attempts to escape dualism in psychiatric theory and practice. As early as 1902, Meyer became disenchanted with neurophysiological explanations of mental illness and elaborated a concept of the individual experiencing unique social and biological influences as "a psychobiological whole" and the view of mental illness as a maladjustment of the entire personality rather than the result of brain pathology [26]. During the 1930s, the so-called psychosomatic movement continued the reaction against 19th century somaticism and neglect of psycho-physical relationships. Originating from psychoanalysis and medicine, psychosomatic medicine focused upon the psychological causes of physical illnesses, enhancing understanding of the role of personality and emotional tensions in disease causation and of the interaction of emotional factors and organic functions [27,28]. Attempting to consider the patient as a whole, to unite "body" and "soul" in medical practice, it extended the prospect of a direct and active psychotherapy intelligently coordinated with the general medical management of the patient.

As psychosomatic medicine and a host of new psychological approaches evolved, so did new physical methods of treatment. Neuropsychiatry received new impetus from the biomedical sciences early in the century. Advances in microbiology demonstrated that infectious agents could attack the central nervous system and produce serious psychiatric disturbances. Increased understanding of nutritional deficiency diseases revealed that vitamin deficiencies may cause disorders such as pellagra and beri-beri, which affect brain metabolism and result in psychotic symptoms. Advances in biochemistry and genetics and knowledge of inborn errors of metabolism clarified the basis of phenylketonuria and the attendant mental retardation. There was increasing knowledge of endocrine interactions and reported favorable effects of thyroid extracts on cretinous patients. All developments fueled the expectation that the physiological basis of mental illness would be understood and made accessible to effective therapy. Appropriate models of organic mental illness and organic therapy of psychotic conditions were generated, and, simultaneously, the increasing recognition of the interaction of biodynamic factors initiated a shift in emphasis from morphological pathology toward fundamental biodynamic interrelations and the multifactoral etiology of disease.

New theories, emphases, and hopes notwithstanding, the psychiatric physical treatment methods introduced before mid-century were of empirical derivation. The first successful physical method of treatment was fever therapy, applied in cases of general paresis, the first psychosis of known organic basis [29]. This encouraged development of other physical methods for the functional psychoses, and shock therapy became popular. It was not a novel approach—artificial shock was used as a treatment method since antiquity—but it was of novel form. The first modern shock therapy, insulin coma therapy, was introduced in the 1930s [30], and a convulsive method using cardiazol appeared soon thereafter

[31]. Electro-shock began to replace cardiazol as a convulsant technique after 1938, at about the same time psychosurgery was introduced [32, 33].

PSYCHOPHARMACOLOGY AND PROSPECTS OF COMBINED THERAPY

Earlier somatic techniques now appear to be superseded by advances in psychopharmacology. Like shock therapy, drugs have long been used to treat mental disorders. A strong scientific interest in psychotropic drugs emerged in the mid-19th century, and opiates, chloral hydrate, bromides, barbiturates, alcohol, and caffeine were used extensively thereafter. During the 1930s, amphetamine derivatives and sodium amytal were commonly employed, and narcotherapy, utilizing barbiturates and carbon dioxide, was practiced throughout the 1940s, especially in treatment of traumatic war neuroses. Historically, however, the general pattern of drug therapy has been one of initial enthusiasm followed by disappointment. Witness the history of the bromides. Soon after their discovery in 1826, bromides were widely used in treatment of psychiatric illnesses. Their use increased late in the century, when it was found that they relieved uncontrollable states of excitement. By the mid-1920s, some claimed that finally a drug was available that could alleviate serious symptoms of disturbed behavior, and in 1928 every fifth prescription was for bromides [34]. But as clinical data accumulated, great expectations yielded to disillusionment and bromide use receded in psychiatric practice.

Disappointments notwithstanding, the search for effective psychoactive medications continued. Before mid-century, most drugs used in psychiatric treatment were sedatives, and many calmed the patients temporarily by rendering them unconscious. In the continued quest for therapeutic psychotropic drugs, there was the hope for drugs that would tranquilize patients without depriving them of consciousness or inducing a state of confusion. It was the introduction of such drugs during the decade after World War II that established modern psychopharmacology and dramatically changed the treatment of mental illness.

For centuries the snakeroot plant was used in India to treat a variety of maladies ranging from snakebite to insanity, and it was known to produce contentment without cloudiness. The West

learned of the plant in the 17th century, when it was named
Rauwolfia serpentina. However, its medical potential was unrecognized until 1931 [35] and was not exploited until after 1952, when
the alkaloid reserpine was isolated from its roots and found to be
effective in treating hypertension and psychoses without significantly impairing consciousness, memory, or intellectual functioning.
Another antipsychotic drug, chlorpromazine, evolved through laboratory investigation and appeared in 1952 [36]. Soon thereafter,
meprobomate was introduced as an effective antianxiety drug [37].
At about the same time, it was observed that an antitubercular drug
isoniazid appeared to relieve depression [38], and the resultant search
for a less toxic antidepressant led to the introduction of monoamine
oxidase inhibitors and imipramine. During a remarkably brief period,
four new types of therapeutic drugs were entered into practice and
broad new horizons opened in psychiatry. The use of psychotropic
drugs helped to shorten the hospital stay and simplify management
of seriously disturbed patients, reduced the use of more drastic
methods of treating psychotics, enhanced the deinstitutionalization
of psychiatry, and significantly affected office practice.

Pharmacology is the most recent incarnation of the organic
approach in psychiatry extending from Griesinger through Kraepelin.
Psychotherapy, whose genealogy embraces Mesmer, Bernheim, and
Freud, also thrives within contemporary psychiatry and includes non-medical models, practices, and personnel undreamt of a century ago.
The two approaches coexist but do not necessarily cohabit, reflecting
in part the historic separation of somatic and psychological
approaches stemming from the "mind-body" dichotomy dominating
Western thought since the medieval period. The mind-body problem
endures and defies easy resolution because it derives from a fundamental concept of man rooted more in philosophy and theology than
in medicine. Yet it underlies the basic question of the reality of
mental illness and appropriate therapy and mandates definition of
mental causation and mental disease as a theoretical category distinct
from physical disease calling for unique treatment, eg, psychotherapy. In the meantime, however, it is necessary to tend the
garden, and an integrated medical and psychological approach has
begun to evolve in clinical psychiatry through the union of psychotherapy and pharmacotherapy [39]. Combined therapy doesn't
confront dualism directly, but it does bridge the organic and the
psychological; treatment modalities combining psychoactive medication with psychotherapy offer not only practical promise but represent
a step toward unification of "body" and "soul" in psychiatric practice.

REFERENCES

1. Augustine A: *The Confessions of Saint Augustine*, translated by Pusey E. New York: Modern Library, 1949
2. Aquinas T: *Saint Thomas Aquinas, Philosophical Texts*, translated by Gilby T. New York: Oxford University Press, 1960
3. Sprenger J, Kramer H: *Malleus Maleficarum*. London: Folio Society, 1968
4. Weyer J: *De praestigiis daemonum*. Basileae: J Oporinum, 1563
5. Descartes R: Meditations on first philosophy. In *The Philosophical Works of Descartes*, vol 1, edited by Haldane E, Ross G. Cambridge: Cambridge University Press, 1968
6. Locke J: *An Essay Concerning Human Understanding*. Chicago: Henry Regery, 1956
7. Condillac E: Traité des sensations. In *Oeuvres Philosophiques de Condillac*, edited by Le Roy G. Paris: Presses Universitaire de France, 1947
8. Pinel P: *Nosographie philosophique ou la méthode de l'analyse appliqué à la médecine*. Paris: Brosson, 1798
9. Pinel P: *Traité médico-philosophique sur l'alienation mentale*. Paris: Brosson, 1801
10. Connolly J: *An Enquiry Concerning the Indications of Insanity*. London: John Taylor, 1830
11. Holland H: *Chapters on Mental Physiology*. London: Churchill, 1858
12. Griesinger W: *Die Pathologie und Therapie der psychischen Krankheiten*. Stuttgart: Krabbe, 1845
13. Romberg M: *Lehrbuch der Nervenkrankheiten des Menschen*. Berlin: Duncker, 1846
14. Meynert T: *Psychiatrie. Klinik der Erkankungen des Vorderhirns*. Wien: Braumüller, 1884
15. Westphal C: *Psychiatrische Abhandlungen*. Berlin: Hirschwald, 1892
16. Kraepelin E: *Compendium der Psychiatrie*. Leipzig: Abel, 1883
17. Dunn R: *An Essay on Physiological Psychology*. London: Churchill, 1858
18. Maudsley H: *Responsibility in Mental Disease*. London: Kegan Paul, 1874
19. Mesmer F: *Mémoire sur la découverte du magnétisme animal*. Genève, Paris: Didot le jeune, 1779
20. Puységur A-M-J de: *Mémoires pour servir á l'histoire et à l'éstablissement du magnétisme animal*, 2nd ed. Paris: Collot, 1809
21. Braid J: *Neurypnology, or the Rationale of Nervous Sleep Considered in Relation with Animal Magnetism*. London: Churchill, 1843
22. Beard G: *A Practical Treatise on Nervous Exhaustion (Neurasthenia)*. New York: Wood, 1880
23. Charcot J: *Oeuvres complètes, Lecons sur les maladies du système nerveux*. Paris: Progreés Médical, 1890
24. Liébault A: *Du sommeil et des états analgues considérés surtout au point du vue de l'action du moral sur le physique*. Paris: Masson, 1866
25. Bernheim H: *Hypnotisme, suggestion, psychothérapie, Etude Nouvelles*. Paris: Doin, 1891
26. Meyer A: *Collected Works of Adolf Meyer*, edited by Winters E, Bowers A. Baltimore: Johns Hopkins Press, 1950–1952

27. Heyer G: *Das Körperlich-Seelische Zusammenwirken in den Lebensvorgängen.* Munich: Bergman, 1925
28. Bellak L (ed): *Psychology of Physical Illness: Psychiatry Applied to Medicine, Surgery and the Specialties.* New York: Grune and Stratton, 1952
29. Wagner-Jaurreg J: Ueber die Einwirkung fieberhafter Erkrankungen auf Psychosen. *Jb Psychiat* 7:94-134, 1887
30. Sakel M: Schizophreniebehandlung mittels Insulin-Hypoglykämie sowie hypoglykämischer Shocks. *Wien Med Wochenschr* 84: 1211-1214, 1934
31. Meduna L: Versuche über die biologische Beeinflussung des Ablaufes der Schizophrenie. 1. Campher-und Cardiazolkrämpfe. *Z Ges Neurol Psychiat* 152:235-262, 1935
32. Cerletti U: Un nuovo metodo di shockterapia: "L'elettroshock." *Bol R Accad Med Roma* 64:136-138, 1938
33. Moniz E: Prefrontal leucotomy in the treatment of mental disorder. *Am J Psychiatry* 93:1379-1385, 1936
34. Wright W: Results obtained by the intensive use of bromides in functional psychoses. *Am J Psychiatry* 5:365-389, 1926
35. Sen G, Bose K: *Rawolfia serpentina*, a new Indian drug for insanity and high blood pressure. *Indian Med World* 2:194-201, 1931
36. Delay J, Deniker P: Trent-huit cas de psychoses traitées par la cure prolongée et continue de 4560 R. P. *C R Congr Alien et Neurol de Langue Franc* Paris: Masson, 1952
37. Berger F: The pharmacological properties of 2-methyl-2-m-propyl-1, e-propanediol dicarbomate (Miltown), a new interneuronal blocking agent. *J Pharmacol* 112:413-423, 1954
38. Flaherty J: The psychiatric use of isonicotinic acid hydrazine: A case report. *De Med J* 24:198-201, 1952
39. Karasu T: Psychotherapy and pharmacotherapy: Toward an integrated model. *Am J Psychiatry* 139:1102-1113, 1982

CHAPTER 2

Ideologic Conflicts in Combined Treatment

Gerald L. Klerman

PSYCHIATRIC SCHOOLS AS IDEOLOGIES

The topic of combined treatment is a timely one. There is increasing utilization of mental health services by the population and a growing acceptance by professionals and the public of pharmacotherapy and psychotherapy, alone and in combination.

However, discussion of issues of psychiatric treatment with laymen and professionals soon leads to the awareness that the attitudes, expectations, and perceptions of the discussants are heavily determined by their commitments to ideological positions. Thus, patients often say, "My therapist doesn't believe in drugs." In contrast, biologically oriented psychiatrists will say "I don't believe in psychotherapy, it's just paying for friendship." These conflicting attitudes toward psychotherapy and pharmacotherapy are reflections of larger sources of conflict and strain within the American mental health field.

THE SCHOOLS OF PSYCHIATRY

Various distinct emphases emerged early in the relatively brief history of psychiatry in the United States for the study and treatment of mental disorder—the biological organism, mental processes (the conscious and unconscious), the societal and institutional setting for care, and socially adaptive behavior. While the dominance of one or several of these emphases fluctuated in different historic eras for differing social and historical reasons, these emphases have provided the basis for the growth of multiple, competing psychiatric schools, each of which, in turn, has developed a particular theoretical research and treatment framework.

It is important to recognize that at the present time no school is dominant in the United States. The psychiatric profession currently has many scientific sources, drawing on specialized knowledge within its own broad sphere, ranging from psychoanalysis to psychobiology, as well as related disciplines of psychology and epidemiology. The diversity characterizing the professional scene has resulted in considerable ferment, competition, and rivalry among the alternative schools. The extent of this diversity has been described by Armor and Klerman [1], Havens [2], and Lazare [3].

Observers of the American scene have catalogued the diverse schools in various ways. In their influential study of social class and mental illness, Hollingshead and Redlich [4] divided the practitioner community in New Haven into two groups, which they named the Analytic and Psychological (A-P) and Directive and Organic (D-O). Subsequent researchers described other groupings. In the early 1960s, Strauss and his associates in Chicago [5], using sociological survey methods, and Armor and Klerman [1], studying a nationwide sample of psychiatrists working in hospitals, identified three psychiatric schools: a biological (or organic) school, a psychological/psychodynamic school, and what was then emerging as a social psychiatric school.

During the 1960s and 1970s, there was a proliferation of new therapies, both psychosocial and biological, and new ideas and points of views. Psychiatrists and other mental health professionals grew in number and in public recognition. Utilization of mental health services, both public and private, expanded rapidly, such that by 1980, about 10 percent of the adult population saw a mental health professional in a year.

Table 1 describes the five major psychiatric schools most relevant to psychiatric treatment in general, and the issues of combined treatment in particular.

Table 1. Contemporary Schools of Psychiatry

School	Major US Proponents	Theoretical Sources	Applications and Emphases
Biological	Kety Winokur E. Robins	19th century Continental medical thought	Pharmacotherapy Genetic studies Central nervous system research
Psychoanalytic	Erikson Kohut Kernberg	Freudian psychoanalytic concepts and American modifications, particularly ego psychology and self-psychology	Intensive, insight-oriented psychotherapy and psychoanalysis
Interpersonal	Sullivan Fromm-Reichmann Arieti	Social and developmental psychology	Broadened psychotherapeutic framework to include family and group therapies Psychotherapy with schizophrenia, depression, and other severe conditions
Social	Meyer Leighton Lindemann	Sociology, anthropology, and other social sciences	Epidemiologic studies Community mental health
Behavioral	Wolpe Stunkard Beck	Pavlovian and Skinnerian learning theory Cognitive psychology	Behavior therapies Cognitive therapy

Observers of the American scene will note that a number of influential groups of practitioners are not represented here. For example, an existential school, identified and described by Havens [2], has influenced many modern thinkers and writers by extending tenets of existential philosophy and literature into therapeutic theory, but has had relatively little impact on psychiatric research or practice. Schools of psychotherapy that have proliferated in the last decade, particularly among nonmedical practitioners (such as Gestalt therapy, humanistic psychology, and transactional analysis), have often been hostile to the "medical model" in psychiatry and its modes of diagnosis and classification. The community mental health movement also does not appear here as a separate school; although it has effected major changes in the delivery of mental health services, its theoretical basis lies in social psychiatry and much of its clinical practice uses interpersonal approaches. The theoreticians and practitioners of community health are, in fact, often critical of the "medical model" and often are allied in an antidiagnostic stance with the "antipsychiatry movement."

Schools as Ideologies

Reference to schools of psychiatry in the United States focuses on internal divisions reflecting the different beliefs and cognitive views within the mental health professions. However, the ideas and views of these various schools are held strongly by their proponents, so much so that discussion of scientific and professional issues among psychiatrists and mental health professionals is often attended by dispute, dissension, and acrimony. To further describe the complexity of the American psychiatric scene, the sociological concept of "ideology" is useful.

Although most prominently explored and applied in the fields of social, economic, and political theory [6], the concept of ideology has been extended to understanding the processes of cohesion and fragmentation in professions [1,5].

A professional ideology consists of four components:

1. *Cognitive.* This component refers to the theories, ideas, and beliefs regarding the nature of the field and the major aspects.

2. *Prescriptive or Normative.* The ideas comprise not only what *is*—what exists in the field—but also judgments as to norms, what *should be* applied to clinical practice, teaching, and research.

3. *Emotive.* Emotional and attitudinal components are attached to the ideas and beliefs. The beliefs are held strongly by

each school's adherents, often with conviction, zeal, and determination.

4. *Social and Affiliative.* Members of each school seek each other out, leading to the formation of and participation in informal groups and professional organizations, such as societies and associations.

These four components often combine and result in psychiatric schools becoming "movements," involving not only the members of the profession but intellectuals, journalists, legislators, and others outside the profession allied with a school's particular views. Thus, we identify a "psychoanalytic movement" or a "community mental health movement," whereas for other fields of medicine we would seldom, if ever, refer to a "surgical movement" or a "cancer movement."

The schools of American psychiatry have differed strongly as to their concepts of mental illness, as well as on specific aspects of diagnostic reliability and validity, and appropriateness of treatment. The differences between the schools also extend to moral and ethical judgments; some schools, for example, regard diagnostic efforts as depersonalizing and antitherapeutic and, at times, politically repressive.

THE IMPACT OF IDEOLOGY UPON THE RESPONSE TO NEW PSYCHOPHARMACOLOGIC AGENTS IN THE 1950s AND 1960s

With the introduction of drug therapy in the mid-1950s, American psychiatrists and other mental health professionals were divided in their attitudes toward the value of drugs in the treatment of mental conditions, whether alone or in combination with psychotherapy. In retrospect, it is possible to identify four groups of clinicians: the proponents of drug therapy, the skeptics, the radical critics, and the pragmatic combiners. I herein review the points of view expressed by members of these four groups and critically analyze the ideological bases for their response.

The Proponents of Drug Therapy

Many psychiatrists argue in favor of a causal relationship between the introduction of modern drug therapy and the improvements that occurred during the treatment of the mentally ill, particularly those

hospitalized with psychotic states but also the ambulatory psychoneurotic patients. This view was most widely held by biological
psychiatrists and by mental health professionals working in public
mental health institutions with severely ill patients, but was also
advanced by a large number of practitioners in private settings and
outpatient clinics who belong to what Hollingshead and Redlich [4]
identified as the "directive and organic" group of practitioners.
These psychiatrists, along with many journalists and public officials,
concluded that the new drugs not only improved patient treatment
but brought about a revolution in psychiatry, putting psychiatry
back into the "mainstream" of modern medicine. Many proponents
of drug therapy have an implicit, at times exquisite, antipsycho-
therapeutic bias and regard the success of drug therapy as support for
their long-held criticism of Freudianism and related psychotherapeutic theories. The early proponents of pharmacotherapy of depression included many former advocates of electroconvulsive therapy
(ECT) and adherents of lithium, such as Kline [7] and Fieve [8],
who often combined their support of ECT and drug therapy with
criticism of psychotherapy as being of limited value, at best.

The Skeptics

The skeptics comprise private practitioners skilled in psychotherapy, and a large group of social psychiatry researchers who
questioned whether the new tranquilizers and related drugs had any
"real" effect. They agreed that psychiatry had witnessed periods of
enthusiasm and optimism for such new treatments as mesmerism in
the 18th century, moral treatment and phrenology in the 19th
century, and numerous other fads for both psychic and somatic
treatments. The skeptics pointed to the extensive research in indus-
trial settings on the Hawthorne effect, whereby any increase in attention and enthusiasm had a positive effect on a group situation,
ameliorating conflict and increasing the productivity of workers.
The skeptics wondered if similar enthusiasm and attention on the
part of previously pessimistic and nihilistic physicians could be
communicated to patients and their families. This Hawthorne effect
of clinician's zeal would then interact positively with the placebo
effect of the patient's participation and expectations. Perhaps the
therapeutic benefits attributed to drugs were the result of social-
psychological forces rather than the pharmacologic actions of the
drugs on the central nervous system.

The Radical Critics

While the skeptics raised questions, the radical critics openly condemned these drugs. They argued that not only were the drugs little more than placebo, but, more importantly, that they were actually detrimental to the patient's welfare and had adverse effects on the patient, the psychiatrists, and the family. Drug therapy impaired the patient's progress in psychotherapy by increasing reliance on biological treatment, fostering dependency on the physician, and blunting capacity for insight. In addition to these deleterious effects, the new tranquilizing drugs were regarded as having even more harmful effects on psychotherapists, limiting their skill by their latent tendencies to find quick solutions to complex social problems. Similar concerns were expressed about the family who would see drug treatment as an explanation of the patient's illness in terms of "nerves" and "real illness," rather than face the conflict, guilt, and other psychological issues that may involve personal responsibility and the need for change in lifestyle or family practices. The radical critics challenged the medical approach as being authoritarian and biological, and stated that in prescribing drugs, physicians used chemical straightjackets or participated in the maintenance of conformity in this repressive society.

Implicit in this viewpoint is the concept of "negative placebo effect." Feminist therapists come closest to expressing this point of view concerning the treatment of depression. They propose that pharmacotherapy hinders "true feminist" psychotherapy because it regards the depressed woman's problems as biomedical and deflects the patient's attention from consciousness-raising efforts and ultimately from social change that would end sexism and promote equality.

The Pragmatic Combiners

The largest group of practitioners have been eclectic and pragmatic. Whatever their theoretical orientation, in practice they have prescribed drugs with increasing frequency. They often combine drugs with psychotherapy on a trial-and-error basis, but the theoretical justifications for this practice remain vague.

By prescribing drugs in combination with the psychotherapy of depression, psychiatrists expect the drugs to reduce manifest symptoms and lower the subjective distress of the patient. Such prominent symptoms as anxiety, insomnia, tension, and autonomic nervous system irregularities became the targets for drug prescription. The psychiatrist hopes thereby to facilitate communication, to reduce resistance to therapeutic insight, and to accelerate psychotherapeutic progress.

THE CURRENT SCENE: THE IMPACT OF ADVANCES IN PSYCHOPHARMACOLOGY ON THE IDEOLOGICAL SCHOOL

In the three decades since the introduction of chlorpromazine, many other chemical classes of compounds with diverse therapeutic actions have appeared. The efficacy of most of these new drugs has been established by controlled studies and their utilization in clinical practice has expanded.

Drugs and psychotherapy are derived from different theoretical realms and should be neutral toward each other, but ideologically they are competitive. The literature of two decades ago was not concerned with the efficacy of psychotherapy in mental disorders compared with or in combination with drug therapies, but mainly questioned how and when, if at all, drugs should be introduced into the psychotherapeutic treatment of patients. These questions reflected the ideologic dominance of psychoanalysis and other forms of psychotherapy at that time.

With increased acceptance of pharmacotherapy for psychiatric disorders, the direction of concern about the effects of drugs on psychotherapy reversed to include questions about the influence of psychological factors on drug treatment.

As the nature of the many forms of psychotherapy was clarified and as evidence for the drug therapies accumulated, more sophisticated hypotheses about the interactions of drugs and psychotherapy as combined treatments were developed. In addition to the originally postulated detrimental effects of adding drugs to psychotherapy, the effects were seen as going in either direction—effects of drugs on psychotherapy or psychotherapy on drugs. Furthermore, the interactions between treatments were seen as being potentially positive as well as negative.

In the 1950s, the focus changed dramatically. With the growing volume of double-blind randomized studies on the efficacy of various forms of pharmacotherapy and the reevaluation of electroconvulsive therapy, scientific judgement has increasingly questioned the nature of the evidence for the value of psychotherapy. The discrepancy between ideology and evidence in psychotherapy has now become the subject of professional and public debate.

These ideologic differences are reflected in clinical practice. Within psychiatry, there is divergence based upon theoretical allegiance. Thus, self-identified biologic therapists "do not believe" in psychotherapy and communicate such attitudes to their patients. Conversely, many psychotherapeutically oriented psychiatrists "do not believe" in drug therapy or disparage it as being "only a crutch," or "only symptom reduction," and they communicate these attitudes to their patients. To complicate the situation further, the large and growing number of nonmedical mental health professionals—psychologists, social workers, psychiatric nurses, pastoral counselors, marriage and family therapists—who are not trained in psychobiology and psychopharmacology and who legally cannot prescribe medication are often, although not universally, critical or skeptical about the possible value of medication.

These differences within the mental health professions are paralleled by corresponding differences in attitude and expectation among the lay public. A considerable segment of the public, particularly the better-educated middle class groups, have a strong psychological orientation toward emotional and mental problems and come to treatment expecting and wanting psychological explanations for their disorders and are skeptical of the value of medication.

However, with the growing evidence for the efficacy of pharmacotherapy, significant numbers of the population have come to see their depressions as due to "chemical" imbalance and often seek medication alone or in combination with psychotherapy or counseling. In fact, within some circles, the use of lithium has become a form of social status and the stigma of affective illness has lessened to a degree unexpected perhaps two or three decades ago.

At this point, it is of interest to relate the response of the individual ideological schools to the impact of psychopharmacology.

The *biological psychiatry* ideology has benefited the most from the advances in psychopharmacotherapy. After decades of professional and public decline, the biological school is currently in a period of considerable optimism and confidence. It is interesting to reconstruct how this situation came about. Biological psychiatry had considerable success toward the end of the 19th century. Its greatest achievements were the dramatic demonstration that central nervous system syphilis was caused by Treponema pallidum and that pellagra was due to vitamin deficiency. After the 1920s, there followed decades of new scientific discoveries in biological psychiatry,

paralleled by a period of excess therapeutic enthusiasm for procedures such as colectomy, excision of teeth, adrenalectomy,
intravenous metrozol for convulsive treatment, and prefrontal
lobotomy. Often these treatments were introduced with minimum
attention to scientific evidence and with lack of attention to the
need for informed consent. Many observers, both within the professions and the public-at-large, were appalled by what they felt were
indiscriminate application of brutalizing treatments derived from
fanciful theories and based on insufficient evidence as to their
efficacy and safety. Although the adherents of biological psychiatry
are relatively few in number, representing only a minority of psychiatrists or psychiatric practitioners, the quality of research and the
influence of basic knowledge upon practice has increased. Among
the academic psychiatrists, the biological psychiatry ideology is the
major source of research activity; this approach has the most support
among other physicians and among the majority of the public,
including policymakers. Within the biological psychiatry group, there
is a strong antipathy to psychotherapy, which is reflected often in
extreme depreciation of its possible value and often in higher thresh-
olds for the acceptance of evidence as to efficacy and safety.

Among *psychoanalysts and psychoanalytically oriented psychotherapists*, the impact of psychopharmacology has been considerable.
Professionally dominant in the 1950s and early 1960s, psychodynamic psychotherapy and psychoanalysis is now on the defensive.
Although most psychiatric and other mental health professionals
identify themselves as dynamic psychotherapists, intellectually and
scientifically this ideology is on the decline. It is notable that a
number of psychoanalysts have made attempts to integrate pharmacotherapy oriented psychotherapy. Notable among this group are
Mortimer Ostow in New York, G. Sarwer-Foner in Canada, and
Lewis Gottschalk in California. In practice, the majority of
psychiatrists identify themselves as "eclectic," which means that they
start from a dynamic psychotherapeutic base and add behavioral,
interpersonal, and drug therapy on a pragmatic case-by-case basis.
It is to this group that the research reported in this volume may have
the greatest impact.

Behavioral ideology emerged in the 1960s based upon the
learning theories of Skinner and Pavlov. At first, its major adherents
were among psychologists and during the militant phase, issues
revolving around the relative efficacy of behavioral therapy versus
other techniques of psychotherapy were mixed with the struggles
between psychologists and psychiatrists.

It is of note that the two new treatments introduced in the 1960s, behavior therapies and psychopharmacologic treatments, made extensive use of the randomized control trial. These new treatments tried to challenge the dominant ideology, then represented by psychoanalysis, and resorted to evidence from controlled studies to buttress their position. Behavioral techniques are gradually being diffused into psychiatry, particularly psychosomatic medicine and behavioral medicine. There have been systematic attempts to study the interaction between drugs and behavioral techniques in eating disorders and phobias.

The *interpersonal school* has had considerable difficulty accepting the role of medication, particularly those interpersonal psychotherapists who worked closely with schizophrenic patients utilizing the teachings of Fromm-Reichmann and the group at Chestnut Lodge. Psychotherapy alone for hospitalized psychotic schizophrenic patients is ineffective. Of the seven controlled studies, only one shows any possible benefit from psychotherapy alone. Consequently, it appears that the value of interpersonal psychotherapies in schizophrenia occurs only in the presence of concomitant antipsychotic medication.

It is in the area of family therapy, however, that the interpersonal school has had its greatest influences. The combination of medication and family therapy is often hindered by the ideologic position taken by many family systems therapists that there is no patient and there is no disorder but that the problem lies within the system. Given that definition of the problem, it is often difficult for family systems therapists to acknowledge that there is an identified patient with distress and symptoms who meets the criteria of a disorder, such as schizophrenia, drug abuse, depression, and that the symptomatic treatment of that condition in the identified patient will reduce the stress on the family system to a significant degree.

The *social psychiatry* ideology has had major revisions of its ideology, particularly through the 1970s. The community mental health movement arose from within the social psychiatry movement and increasingly has taken on a radical wing. The "radical" social ideology is anti-medical, anti-biological, anti-diagnostic and anti-institutional. It sees the problems of mental patients as not residing within the patient, but rather the patient as a victim of a repressive, racist, sexist, and exploitative society. Within this point of view, medications are anathema and the adverse effects of phenothiazines as manifested in movement disorder are often emphasized. The radical ideology also criticizes the use of medication as an extention of social control; this has contributed to the numerous court cases which revolve around whether or not institutionalized patients have the right to refuse treatment.

CLINICAL APPLICATIONS

Having reviewed the ideological conflicts in combined treatment, let us assess how these conflicts influence clinical practice. We shall do this by analyzing a number of hypotheses about the possible interactions—positive and negative—between psychotherapy and pharmacotherapy.

Possible Negative Effects of Drug Therapy on Psychotherapy

Most attention has been paid to the possible negative effects of introducing drug therapy into psychotherapy. Although relatively little empirical research has been done on this problem, it is possible to identify a number of proposed interactions.

Much of the criticism of drug therapy enunciated by psychotherapists in the 1950s implied a negative placebo effect—that pill taking had harmful effects in the presence of psychotherapy. It was hypothesized that the prescription of any drug had deleterious effects upon the psychotherapeutic relationship and upon the attitudes and behavior of both patients and therapist—effects independent of the specific pharmacological actions of the drug. Moreover, the prescription of medication promoted an authoritarian attitude on the part of the psychiatrist and enhanced his belief in his biological-medical heritage. At the same time, the patient would become more dependent, place greater reliance on magical thinking, and assume a more passive, compliant role, as is expected in the conventional doctor-patient relationship in fields of medicine other than psychiatry.

Drug-induced reduction of symptoms as motives for discontinuing psychotherapy In contrast to the negative placebo effect hypothesis earlier, which deals only with the symbolic and psychological meaning of drug administration, another hypothesis acknowledges the pharmacological and therapeutic actions of drugs, but expresses concern lest the resultant decrease of the patient's anxiety and tension reduce motivation for psychotherapeutic participation. The hypothesis predicts that too effective a drug will initiate forces operating counter to psychotherapy. Thus, if a psychoactive drug, such as a phenothiazine or diazepoxide derivative, is highly effective in reducing psychotic turmoil, neurotic anxiety, or other symptoms, the patient's motivation for reflection, insight, and psychotherapeutic work will be lessened. According to this hypothesis, it is predicted that if drug therapy is too effective, patients will no longer seek psychotherapy because they will be satisfied with symptom reduction and therefore cease working toward deeper personality and character changes.

Pharmacotherapy undercuts defenses This hypothesis predicts that if the pharmacological effect of a drug prematurely undercuts some important defenses, symptom substitution or other compensatory mechanisms of symptom formation will ensue. For example, in psychotherapeutic practice, Seitz [9] reported instances of new symptom formation after hypnosis, and Weiss [10] cautioned against an overly rapid relief of the anxiety of the agoraphobic, because if such anxiety is reduced too rapidly, before new defenses are developed, other symptoms may occur. This hypothesis assumes that symptoms maintain a balance between conflict and defenses, and that the precipitous reduction of anxiety, depression, or tension may upset this equilibrium and release deeper conflicts. If so, this disequilibrium would obviously generate new symptoms for the depressive patient; however, systematic research data and replications germane to this specific hypothesis are few and inconclusive.

Possible deleterious effects of pharmacotherapy upon therapy expectations The hypothesis predicts that there may be a negative reaction when the patient is prescribed drug therapy instead of psychotherapy, if he/she expected the latter. Patients may feel that the prescription of a drug defines them as "less interesting," not a candidate for insight. Thus, the use of drugs may initiate a loss of self-esteem on the part of some patients, especially if they belong to a cultural subgroup whose values emphasize insight, psychotherapeutic understanding, and self-actualization. This expectation varies with the social class and subculture in which the patient participates. Within groups that value psychotherapy, the use of drugs is often regarded as a "failure" or a "crutch."

Possible Positive Effects of Drug Therapy on Psychotherapy

The four aforementioned hypotheses describe negative influences
of drugs on the psychotherapeutic process. Although these possible
negative influences have been given the most attention by clinicians,
in a comprehensive analysis equal consideration must be given to the
possible positive effects by which drug therapy may facilitate, augment, and interact in a synergistic manner with psychotherapy and
other therapies. At least four such hypotheses may be identified.

Drugs facilitate psychotherapeutic accessibility   This hypothesis
is embodied in the most commonly stated rationales for the use of
combined therapies, and it supports prevailing clinical practice in
psychiatry. Advertisements and other promotional materials of many
pharmaceutical firms propose that the introduction of their drug
facilitates psychotherapy by making the patient "more accessible."
The proposed mechanism for this effect is readily specified—the
pharmacological action of the drug ameliorates the presumed central
nervous system dysfunction underlying symptom formation, resulting
in reduction of the patient's symptomatology, psychopathology,
and/or affective discomfort. Drug-induced reduction in discomfort
renders the patient better able to communicate in and benefit from
psychotherapy. While some level of anxiety, dysphoria, or symptomatology is believed necessary to provide the "drive" or "motivation"
for participation in psychotherapy, on the other hand this hypothesis
presumes that excessive levels of tension, anxiety, or symptom intensity result in a decrease in the patient's capacity to participate
effectively in psychotherapy.

*Drugs influence the ego psychological functions required for
participation in psychotherapy*   Another hypothesis predicts that
drugs may positively influence the psychotherapeutic process
through their pharmacological action on neurophysiological sub-
strates for the ego functions necessary for psychotherapeutic participation. Some drugs may influence verbal skills, improve cognitive
functioning, improve memory, reduce distraction, and promote
attention and concentration. Because it is widely accepted that
adequate ego functioning is a prerequisite for psychotherapeutic
participation, these psychological functions and abilities are components of the large domain of ego function and enhance the patient's
benefit from participation in psychotherapy.

Drugs promote abreaction Abreaction is one of the basic psychotherapeutic techniques. Breuer and Freud [11] in their studies of hysteria, describe the use of hypnosis to promote catharsis or abreaction. A number of drugs, especially intravenous barbiturates and amphetamines, have been used to promote this effect. Wikler [12], in his monograph on the pharmacological basis of psychiatric therapy, referred to such methods as "psychoexploratory" techniques. These drugs help to uncover memory, break down defenses, and bring into consciousness material against which the person otherwise defends. A variant of this practice is the use of LSD, mescaline, and psilocybin to promote "peak experiences" in which the heightened sense of self-awareness and emotional, affective, and bodily experiences that occur under these psychedelic drugs are advocated as facilitating the psychotherapeutic process.

Positive effect of drug therapy on expectation and stigma In addition to the short-term symptomatic relief of drug therapy, a positive placebo effect may often contribute to a general attitude of optimism and confidence on the part of the patient. The advocates of biological methods, such as the megavitamin treatment of schizophrenia, are, in effect, removing some of the stigma from psychiatric illness and are in some instances making it easier for the patients to accept the definition of themselves as being mentally ill. Thus, the request for drug therapy may itself be a vehicle through which the patient can seek psychotherapeutic help and counseling. In this sense, the skillful psychiatrist often uses the patient's initial request for drug therapy as a starting point for initiating a psychotherapeutic process.

Possible Negative Effects of Psychotherapy Upon Drug Therapy

Most of the discussion in the literature has focused on possible effects of drug therapy upon psychotherapy. Relatively little attention has been paid to the other side of the process, namely, the impact of psychotherapy upon the patient receiving pharmacotherapy. It is interesting to note how seldom this problem is discussed or even mentioned.

Perhaps, considering the demonstrated efficacy of drugs for the treatment of affective disorders and the relatively less extensive body of evidence for the efficacy of psychotherapy, the question should be stated: What negative effects or benefits accrue to the patient if psychotherapy is added to drug therapy? During the discussions in

the 1950s and 1960s, the psychotherapists were the assertive members of the dialogue, and the drug therapists were on the defensive.
Now one can discern a shift with the impact of evidence as to drug
efficacy from controlled studies.

Biochemical replacement effect of drugs Some pharmacotherapies compare psychotropic drug treatment to the conventional
nonpsychiatric use of drugs in medicine, especially endocrine agents
such as insulin for diabetes. For those who hold this view, the
rectification of the presumed neurophysiological dysfunction
or deficiency is the critical factor, and psychotherapy is considered
unnecessary and irrelevant, or at best neutral. A variation of this
single-factor reductionist hypothesis is expressed by some proponents of lithium treatment of mania. The most extreme version is
proposed by those who advocate megavitamin therapy for schizophrenia. Those holding such views feel that drugs alone are both
necessary and sufficient.

Psychotherapy may be symptomatically disruptive Furthermore,
some pharmacotherapists hypothesize that psychotherapy may be
deleterious to the pharmacological treatment, because symptoms
may be aggravated by excessive probing and uncovering defenses.
Some psychiatrists who work with depressive and schizophrenic
patients feel that harm is done to the patient by psychotherapeutic
intervention, particularly during the acute stage, and that during the
early recovery process the patient is best left alone to "heal over"
and to reconstitute his defenses. There is a clear conflict between
psychiatrists who advocate working through underlying conflicts in
depression and others who support healing over or sealing over
promoting denial, repression, and other defenses. The fear hypothesized by many pharmacotherapists is that psychotherapy, by
uncovering areas of conflict, will increase the levels of tension.
Implicit in this controversy over the validity of this hypothesis may
be the variable of timing: What are the appropriate points in the
process of therapeutic planning at which primarily supportive psychotherapy should be pursued, and when is it appropriate to use
uncovering, probing insight techniques?

Possible Positive Effects of Psychotherapy on Drug Therapy

Psychotherapy as rehabilitation Many drug therapists hypothesize a value for psychotherapy, but in a secondary and ameliorative way. They propose that psychotherapy operates not upon

ideologic mechanisms or upon the core of the psychological process per se, but to correct secondary difficulties in interpersonal relations and in self esteem and psychological functions that follow upon the impact of affective symptoms. In this hypothesis, psychotherapy is seen as rehabilitative rather than as therapeutic in the classical medical model. As such, it would be purely elective rather than a necessary component of the treatment program.

Psychotherapy Facilitates Drug Compliance and Adherence

Psychotherapeutic input (at least at the level of reassurance), personal interest, education and explanation, and clear instructions, will enhance the patient's positive attitude and cooperation.

Philip May and others have distinguished between psychological management and psychotherapy. Psychological management refers to extension of general aspects of doctor-patient relationships to enhance drug compliance and patient cooperation and general therapeutic alliance. Psychotherapy, in this view, refers to efforts to influence the patient's symptoms and psychological functions by verbal and behavioral techniques.

CONCLUSIONS

Reviewing the role of ideology in relation to psychopharmacology and psychotherapy over the past three decades indicates a shift from preoccupations with theoretical preconceptions to attempt to deal with the growing demand for evidence. The ideological schools have had to confront multiple changes, particularly the changing social basis for practice and evidence for the efficacy of various forms of psychotherapy and for multiple forms of pharmacotherapy. In particular, the evidence for the ineffectiveness of psychotherapy alone with schizophrenia and severely depressed patients gives pause to many ideologically committed psychotherapists. In this situation, the value of combined treatment is not only pragmatic in its ability to enhance therapeutic benefit to patients, but also can serve as a valuable moderator upon ideological zeal. Hopefully, the availability of evidence for efficacy of combined therapies in various conditions will lead to cautious attempts at integration of theory and practice.

REFERENCES

1. Armor D, Klerman GL: Psychiatric treatment orientations and professional ideology. *J Health Soc Behav* 9: 243, 1968
2. Havens L: *Approaches to the Mind*. Boston: Little Brown and Co, 1973
3. Lazare A (ed): *Outpatient Psychiatry*. London: Williams and Wilkins, 1979
4. Hollingshead A, Redlich F: *Social Class and Mental Illness*. New York: John Wiley and Co, 1958
5. Strauss A, Schatzman L, et al: *Psychiatric Ideologies and Institutions*. New York: The Free Press, 1964
6. Mannheim K: *Ideology and Utopia*. New York: Harcourt Brace, 1936
7. Kline NS: *From Sad to Glad*. New York: Putnam, 1974
8. Fieve R: *Moodswing: The Third Revolution in Psychiatry*. New York: William Morrow, 1975
9. Seitz PF: Experiments in the substitution of symptoms by hypnosis. *Psychosom Med* 15: 405, 1953
10. Weiss E: Clinical aspects of depression. *Psychoanal Q* 13: 445, 1944
11. Breuer J, Freud S: *Studies in Hysteria*. Boston: Beacon Press, 1950
12. Wikler A: *The Relation of Psychiatry to Pharmacology*. Baltimore: Williams and Wilkins, 1957

PART II

Combined Therapy in Clinical Practice

CHAPTER 3

Psychological Aspects of Medication Management

Nicholas G. Ward

Each aspect of medication management involves psychological issues that deserve attention. Many psychiatrists skilled in managing the psychological issues of psychotherapy do not use these skills when they prescribe medication. Too often, they neglect invaluable psychotherapeutic approaches and use only explanation and admonishment to get patients to take medication. Other clinicians are content to use an intensive bedside manner, a blend of warmth and authority, that is used regardless of the patient's diagnosis or personality. This approach is exemplified in the remarks of an ex-surgeon turned psychiatrist who, in reflecting about his former, highly successful surgical practice, commented that a good physician is "kind, intelligent, and dogmatic."

In this chapter, the focus of the approaches and techniques discussed is on facilitating medication management rather than inducing psychotherapeutic change. The objective is to help patients achieve optimal psychopharmacologic benefits within the context of an optimal patient-physician relationship. May [1] and Epstein and Fawcett [2] offer excellent descriptions of this psychological approach to medication management. Epstein and Fawcett's National Institute of Mental Health (NIMH) manual is devoted entirely to managing depressed patients with antidepressants.

The general goals of medication management include enhancing compliance and the placebo effect while keeping the patient's general welfare in perspective. Sometimes this is a delicate balance. Overzealous and exclusive attention to compliance can interfere with ongoing psychotherapy and with the patient's overall functioning. If a patient is capable of independent action and decisions, it would not be beneficial medication management, for example, to get a patient to take exactly 20 mg of thiothixene a day, tolerate some muscle rigidity, return to weekly appointments exactly on time, and complain very little to the physician. These responses, however, could be regarded as successful compliance.

Although the physician usually does not prescribe a placebo, placebo effects are present also with active medication. These effects can be used to enhance the benefits of the active medication as well as to diminish and, in some cases, to eliminate the benefits or create negative effects (nocebo effect) [3,4]. Too often, the physician regards the placebo effect as something unscientific, magical, and to be ignored in good medication management. Extensive research indicates that the placebo effect is powerful and cannot be eliminated [4]. For these reasons, the physician should not only attend to it in medication management, but also should foster it for optimal effectiveness.

In addition to patient compliance/autonomy and placebo effects, several other important issues in medication management are explored in this chapter. Physicians need to decide what type of relationship they will strive to create, negotiate a treatment agreement that will maximize drug compliance and placebo effects, and consider psychological reactions to dosage, adverse effects, intended effects, and influences from significant others. In addition, the latent content of patient messages may contain important information: transference reactions may impede acceptance, and countertransference reactions may distort proper management. Furthermore, patients who are very negative and/or prone to adverse effects require special approaches.

RELATIONSHIP TYPE:
DIAGNOSTIC AND PERSONALITY VARIABLES

In each patient-physician relationship, the psychopharmacothera-pist must decide how much dependency to allow the patient and how much authority to use with the patient. Chodoff [5] has pointed out, "the time-honored paternalistic model in which two participants are seen, not in a hierarchical stance with each other, but rather as equals negotiating an exchange of technically competent services for financial reimbursement." While recognizing the positive effects of this egalitarian trend, he notes that equal relationships are based on the assumption that the autonomy of participants is intact. Ackerman [6] convincingly argues that illness frequently affects the ability to be autonomous. Thus, paternalism (or maternalism) is not a bad thing per se, but its use or degree of use should be contingent on the patient's inability to function autonomously. To complete matters, Cross and Churchill [7] recommend a "responsible paternalism" that "involves both precise knowledge and empathy to act for the patient on the patient's behalf." Thus, the physician must be able to appreciate the patient's own values and style of living and consider these in making treatment decisions. The physician must choose relationships on a continuum, with one pole being a bene-volent parent-child type of relationship for highly impaired patients and the other pole being a fully collaborative relationship [5,8], for patients who are capable of full autonomy and willing to use it.

The physician must also take into account how much warmth and intimacy the patient can tolerate, the cognitive style of the patient, and the discrepancy between the patient's ability to function autonomously and the patient's perception of his/her autonomy. While warmth has generally been found to be a positive characteristic in a therapist [9], there are some patients who distrust it. The reasons for this distrust may vary from paranoia in a schizophrenic patient, to disbelief in an antisocial personality, to fear of intimacy in a schizoidal or obsessive-compulsive patient. In a review on psycho-therapy with the schizophrenic, McGlashan [10] recommends that the therapist "achieve an optimal distance between closeness and distance in response to patient's ambivalence. The patient is untrust-ing but lonely."

The cognitive style of the patient will further affect how infor-mation is given. Therapists who can match the patient's cognitive style are more likely to give patients information they can use

[11,12] and are more therapeutic [13]. Thus, the obsessive patient will need great detail about medications while the histrionic patient will respond better to more global descriptions [11,12].

The art of psychopharmacotherapy is further challenged by patients who demand far more autonomy than they are capable of, such as grandiose schizophrenics and manics, or by patients who seek far more dependency than they need, such as borderline and histrionic personalities. While all of these principles are fairly obvious, they are frequently not integrated into medication management. It is here that the psychopharmacologist-scientist must merge with the clinician-artist.

How can these principles be translated into clinical practice? With patients capable of little or no autonomy, such as many acute and chronic schizophrenics, a nurturing but firm parent-child relationship is probably appropriate. The physician must be comfortable with giving clear, concrete instructions and advice with supportive but matter-of-fact comments on what the patient is doing. The number of choices these patients must make should be limited so they do not feel overwhelmed, but do feel included in the treatment process. The high degree of authority used in this sort of relationship must always be tempered with a high degree of nurturance. The physician needs to listen empathically to the patient's feelings and experiences as well as to reports bearing psychopharmacologic data.

While a fully egalitarian relationship would probably be a disservice to these patients, the psychopharmacotherapist should be prepared to shift the relationship as the patient improves. As the patient gains more autonomy, the physician needs to allow the patient a wider range of decisions and choices. A nurturant, parental model may still be appropriate as the schizophrenic patient improves, but the therapist can move from acting like the parent of a three-year-old to acting like the parent of a nine-year-old or of an adolescent. Some schizophrenic patients, when given the opportunity, can achieve highly autonomous functioning. In my experience, schizophrenics with high IQs (often paranoid) are capable of abstraction and, when not compromised by florid psychotic processes, can appreciate and use a large range of subtle information in making decisions for themselves.

Narcissistic, dependent, histrionic, and borderline patients as defined in DSM III [14] may misinterpret these young child-parent types of relationships as opportunities to have all their needs met. Managing them is similar to managing a stormy adolescent. In general, the clinician must attempt to develop a relationship midway on both the authority-equality continuum [5] and the warmth-coolness continuum. If limits are needed, great care must be used not to introduce them as if they were expressions of impatience or punishment. Somewhat more nurturance and authority can be used if psychotherapy is not conducted along with medication management. The psychotherapist, however, must regularly challenge the patient's dependency. Global explanation without detail is usually indicated in implementing a treatment plan [11,12] for these patients. All the principles above are much more easily described than implemented. Because such patients' relationships are so highly conflicted, the psychopharmacotherapist's attempts to form a working alliance will be met with great resistance. This endeavor becomes a therapeutic process in itself. Here the clinician cannot just practice medication management.

The compulsive, paranoid, avoidant, and schizoidal patients delineated in DSM III [14] generally require more business-like relationships. Extensive detail and explanation regarding the treatment are reassuring to these patients. While they want their physician to be an expert, they are also more compliant when a number of choices are offered [11,12]. For example, many paranoid patients who balk at taking a fixed dose of an antipsychotic will do better when given a dosage range they can titrate. They might be told to take from 10 to 20 mg of haloperidol: 10 mg per day when they do not feel particularly stressed and up to 20 mg per day when their stress levels are high. Some friendliness is appropriate with these patients, but more warmth may be seen as suspect.

Special care is needed with negative and hostile-dependent patients, the "help-rejecting complainers" [15,16]. These patients often present by asking for extensive advice and complaining about the thorough inadequacy of those who previously treated them. They will appear to be more interested in defeating the physician than in getting better [17]. In addition, hostile patients have been shown to report more adverse effects even to placebos [18]. The usual "I can generally help people and feel hopeful for you" approach of clinicians is frequently disastrous. A more skeptical experimental or paradoxical approach probably will be more effective. Such a patient should be told there is no guarantee of good results and the best that can be offered is an attempt at treatment. The difficulties and side effects involved in treatment should be presented in a matter-of-fact manner. It is reasonable to tell such patients "You will probably have some problems with sedation and dry mouth." If they are devoted to defeating you, they will prove you wrong by minimizing such problems. The skeptical tone should be maintained with the patient after initiating of medication. The patient might be asked, "You are not feeling better yet, are you?" If the patient states that he/she is better, the physician can say, "This seems a bit early for the medication to work." When managed correctly, these patients will defeat the physician by complying with the medication and getting better. At no time should the physician show hopeful excitement in regard to this improvement.

It must be emphasized that these are management and not therapeutic techniques. Such a patient requires extensive psychotherapy to overcome this hostile-dependent style [15,16]. Seriously depressed patients require a much gentler approach since their pessimism outweighs their negativism, and they will agree that the situation is hopeless. Also, not all angry patients are hostile-dependent. The real or transference basis for the anger should be explored and dealt with therapeutically. If the anger is not characterologically based, rapid progress can often be achieved.

The more purely paradoxical approach probably should be used only by those trained and skilled in its application. The therapist should have a good understanding of the patient's defenses and conflicts and should know clearly what function the negativism serves for the patient as he/she interacts with others [19,20]. Only with this information can the therapist hope to formulate a paradox that will help the patient's compliance as well as his/her therapy. A therapist who is angry at the patient should avoid this approach as it can be too easily used as an expression of anger.

TREATMENT AGREEMENT

Every patient started on medications needs an explicit or implicit treatment agreement. This should include some agreement on the nature of the problem(s), a simple explanation of how the medication will work, and instruction in how the treatment will be monitored and adjusted.

Problem Agreement

The patient and the physician must find symptoms that they both agree upon to treat. Too often, the physician assumes that his/her own diagnosis of schizophrenia or depression is enough to begin treatment while the patient does not understand what the diagnosis means or does not agree with it. Most patients present with multiple symptoms, some of which they can agree should be treated. For example, a schizophrenic may state that he hears voices, is aware of plots against him, has difficulty organizing his thoughts, and feels generally anxious. If he firmly believes that the voices and plots are real, he is unlikely to regard them as symptoms for which medication should be used. The physician may consider these the most important symptoms and yet would err by attempting to make these the focus of a treatment agreement. The same paranoid patient may readily accept that haloperidol might be useful for his difficulty in thinking and for his anxiety.

Diamond [21] further recommends that concrete terms are more useful than abstract ones, particularly when treating schizophrenic patients. He notes that "decreasing paranoia" is less important to patients than "being less frightened of people." In addition, the patient's own terminology should be used whenever possible. For example, a manic who has been rambling about "cosmic consciousness" may refuse lithium if it is for "mood swings," but may find it useful if it helps with "centering" and "focusing." Any of these symptoms that patient and physician agree upon can form the focus of treatment. It is equally important for the patient to know what symptoms the medications will not treat, such as boredom or anger at family.

In another case, a patient with a diagnosis of depression may present with pain as the chief complaint and deny depressed mood. Anhedonia and a wide variety of vegetative symptoms might confirm the diagnosis and indicate an antidepressant trial, but a pain patient might resist the idea of taking antidepressants. However, patient and physician can frequently agree that the insomnia, fatigue, anxiety, and pain are symptoms that medications might help. Such a patient can accept that antidepressants are capable of treating these symptoms, but will not accept that he/she is depressed. This can be the basis of a very workable treatment agreement.

Sometimes a treatment agreement will not be possible, yet adequate treatment may be. Some psychotic patients cannot commit themselves to a yes or no answer to anything. To attempt a definite agreement may jeopardize the minimal therapeutic leverage the physician already has. The following case demonstrates one possible approach to this problem.

Case 1. Mr. B., a 25-year-old single man with a six-year history of chronic schizophrenia, was referred from the state hospital to our medication clinic for follow-up depot fluphenazine administration. He had been very unreliable about taking oral medication and had relapsed often. While committed to the hospital, he had been easy to manage. He appeared at the medication clinic close to the appointed time for his injection, but said he was not sure about having the injections. Further inquiry revealed that he was having no adverse effects from the fluphenazine and that he was considerably more functional since starting it. He was not negative, but rather vague and noncommital. We then instituted an approach that was alternately referred to as the "schizophrenic contract" or the "no contract-contract" in our clinic. The patient was told that we needed to give him his injection first and then we needed to talk to him about his other concerns. He did not refuse the injection, but told us afterwards he was not sure he needed to take it. Mr. B. was then given another appointment and advised that we would further discuss his concerns at that point. He again came to the appointment on time, stating that he was not sure about this treatment. The second session was conducted identically to the first with the same results.

Throughout the following year, Mr. B. came to our clinic weekly, but always stated that he was not sure about taking medication. He had no relapses or adverse effects during this year, and he was adjusting adequately to life outside the state hospital.

In this case, it would have been a mistake to try to get agreement on the problem and then to get agreement on treatment. Verbally, he could not agree to treatment, but nonverbally he could. This provided the basis for our "schizophrenic contract." The process was too predictable to consider that the patient was tricked into treatment. If anything, the patient may have felt that he had tricked us by never agreeing to be treated.

Treatment Explanation

The idea that biochemical mechanisms can influence psychological processes is confusing and alien to many patients. Similarly, many other patients find it difficult to believe that psychological processes could affect their disease. These patients are looking for the magic pill. Patients who have an understanding of their disease and its treatment will adhere "more readily" to the treatment process [22,23]. An explanation should be simple and should attempt to integrate biological and psychological mechanisms. Too often, patients who accept simple biochemical imbalance models use them to avoid exploring social and psychological issues and to abdicate responsibility for their actions. The result is a patient who is likely to say "The chemicals made me do it" (rather than the devil) and who will engage the psychopharmacologist in endless searches for better medications to combat the problems of being human.

A more useful explanation might include telling patients that biochemical imbalances leave them more prone to develop pathology (depression, psychosis, mania, etc) under stress. They can be told that medications will help correct the imbalance, but that further work on handling stress might help also. This would leave open the possibility of psychotherapeutic work along with medication. These explanations should be tailored to each patient's explanatory model or personal theory of disease [24]. Explanations that fit with the patient's experience are particularly useful. Many schizophrenic patients can accept that they have a biochemical imbalance and further that this leaves them overly sensitive to their environment (the perceptual filter model of schizophrenia). The following case example illustrates the application of some of these ideas.

Case 2. Mr. M., a 43-year-old married man with a 20-year history of paranoid schizophrenia, was referred for "medication management." While haloperidol was quite effective in treating his psychotic symptoms, he had been hospitalized at least yearly because he would stop taking the medication and would become psychotic. Mr. M. was very intelligent and had been attempting to complete a PhD program for the past 15 years, but he had an acute exacerbation of psychosis whenever he tried to teach or whenever he encountered other major stresses.

At the first interview, he wore wraparound mirrored sunglasses and sat in the most distant chair from my desk. After taking a brief psychiatric history, I asked him how he understood his frequent episodes of psychosis. He said he had been told that stress made him go crazy and that he needed to take medication to keep from going crazy. I asked him if this was his own understanding of his illness, and he said "yes" but that it didn't really explain why he went crazy. I told him that many people like himself were overly sensitive to their environments.

They would notice and not be able to tune out traffic sounds or water in the pipes while engaged in conversation. He said that was definitely true for him. I explained to him that under stress this problem of filtering out stimuli was heightened and that this sensitivity applied not only to external events but to thoughts and fantasies in his head. He said that was his experience and that might be why he went crazy. At this point, Mr. M. took off his sunglasses, leaned forward, made good eye contact, and said, "Tell me more." I then described to him how he might be overly sensitive to every nuance with people and that if he noticed nine positive cues and only one negative cue, it was only natural, in the interest of self-protection, to place more importance on the negative cue. He saw how this could lead to paranoia.

We then discussed how medications such as haloperidol could help him filter out stimuli better, but that the important goal would be to achieve a balance between insensitivity and oversensitivity. He said he thought I understood him and his problem. He accepted this model, and we used it frequently during his treatment. He was given flexibility in using 5 to 20 mg of haloperidol per day. Applying the filter model further, he gave himself quiet times when he felt he was becoming overwhelmed. He remained out of the hospital and in good control for at least three years after the introduction of this disease model and the rapport which developed from his acceptance of it.

Medication Instructions

When giving patients instructions, the physician should keep three major goals in mind: clarity, compliance, and enhancement of the pharmacological effect.

Clarity With most patients, the physician needs to use simple terms and avoid sophisticated concepts. Words such as tiring and relaxing might be substituted respectively for sedating and tranquilizing. Patients should frequently be asked if they have any questions, and with patients who appear to be having difficulty understanding, concrete and easily readable instructions are in order [25,26].

The amount of detail presented should vary with the cognitive and personality style of the patient [11,12]. In all cases, enough information must be given to insure adequate safety and compliance with the drug regime. Compulsive and paranoid patients need more detailed information; physicians should present this information first rather than be confronted later with items these patients might have found in a cast-off Physician's Desk Reference. Histrionic patients should be given more global information. For example, compulsive patients might be told that they are being started on an antidepressant which takes three to four weeks of treatment to reach optimal effectiveness; that they have a 70 percent chance of responding to this particular drug; that an antidepressant reverses symptoms of depression, but is not addicting and will not work by making them feel high or drugged. On the other hand, histrionic patients should be told that they ought to be feeling better in three to four weeks with antidepressant medication and that sleep will probably improve even sooner. Specific fears and concerns of histrionic patients can be handled as they appear.

Compliance Medication noncompliance is a major problem in drug treatment; noncompliance rates are reported at 40 to 50 percent [27]. The form can vary between not taking any medication, to taking too little, to irregularly alternating between too much and too little. While studies have explored numerous ways to assess and increase medication compliance, the single best way is to inquire about compliance in an open nonjudgemental manner [28]. Patients can be asked if they are having difficulty following the dosage schedule and if they find themselves missing doses. They can also be asked how often they forget to take their medication and if the medication is not working yet, if they have decided to stop the medication entirely.

A patient who is taking more or less medication than prescribed or is taking it in a different pattern often has very good reason(s). Using this assumption, the physician should begin discussion with the patient [21]. Obvious reasons include adverse effects or a feeling that the medication is not working. Sometimes patients just starting on medication cannot tolerate an open-ended agreement to take medication, but instead find it easier to try the medication for a specified length of time, such as three or four weeks, and then evaluate the results at the end of that time. All the skills of a good therapist are needed for these discussions. The reasons for non-compliance may have many layers, with overt, conscious ones such as "I don't like those side effects" most available, and less conscious ones such as "I do not want to be controlled by you" underneath. In contrast to a psychotherapy approach, the pharmacotherapist generally should focus on the overt, conscious ones.

Enhancing the pharmacological effect   The effects of medication are considerably enhanced for patients who have a good, trusting relationship with a healer who is caring, strong, and positive. In practice, this means that a better outcome may be achieved by spending time with the patient, expressing concern and interest in his/her welfare, and demonstrating a confident, professional manner [18]. Except with very negative patients, the physician should convey both a realistic and optimistic attitude about the treatment. Patients being started on antidepressants can be told that in most cases they can expect their sleep to improve in the first week or 10 days and that the full antidepressant effect will come later. This statement is realistic and therefore should not create false hope, but at the same time it is stated in positive, hopeful terms. Patients who develop an unrealistic hope eventually feel worse because of disappointment.

While phone checkups may appear to be more efficient, spending more time face-to-face with the patient increases the placebo effect [18]. Particularly when the patient begins treatment, the positive effect of actually coming in to see the physician should not be overlooked. As a patient starts to improve, future check-in sessions can be regarded as times to see how quickly he/she is making progress. In general, these suggestions should not be made if the physician does not believe in them. A physician who recommends a treatment, but is doubtful about its outcome, probably should not be the one to prescribe the medication. These negative attitudes can adversely effect the benefits of proven medications [3,4].

SPECIAL PROBLEMS IN MAINTENANCE THERAPY

After feeling better, many patients will conclude that they no longer need the medication. A new treatment agreement is then required. A patient recovering from a single episode of depression will often need to stay on medication for six to eight months and should be informed of the high risk of relapse associated with premature discontinuation [29]. He/she may also wish to avoid extension of medication because of fears of being dependent, fears of being labelled a psychiatric patient, and/or a desire to forget the experience.

Schizophrenic, manic-depressive, or recurrent depressive patients may need to stay on medication indefinitely. This possibility may be mentioned in the beginning of treatment, but a full discussion should be delayed until the patient has experienced some of the benefits of treatment. Since many patients view their medication as a crutch and not as a central necessity, a diabetes model for maintenance may be helpful. People understand that diabetics have a deficiency of insulin and therefore need insulin for life. Generally this need is not viewed in moralistic, strong versus weak terms. Pharmacotherapy patients can be told that their medication has a similar function for them. Psychotherapeutic work is often needed to help the patient adjust to the idea he/she has a lifelong malady.

Patients with chronic or recurrent illnesses will also need to be taught the signs and symptoms of relapse. For example, Herz and Melville [30] have shown that recurring psychosis is often preceded by insomnia, poor concentration, loss of appetite, and increased apathy or depression. Similar symptoms may precede depression relapse. For other patients, the warning symptoms may be idiosyncratic and can be discerned by careful analysis of the events preceding earlier episodes. Just as patients in psychotherapy may need to practice the application of new coping styles, chronically ill medication patients may fail also before they learn when and how to respond to their own warning signs.

Once taught the symptoms of relapse, some patients will test whether the medication is preventing relapse by temporarily stopping their pills. Because depressive, manic, and schizophrenic relapses often do not occur immediately after medication termination, these patients will wrongly conclude that they no longer need medication. Patients on scheduled drug holidays may reach the same conclusion. To prevent this misunderstanding from happening, patients should be informed about the long courses of medication required for preventing relapse.

For patients taking neuroleptics, tardive dyskinesia should be discussed at the same time as maintenance is addressed. Informed consent should include an accurate account of the disability with the goal of prevention. The patient can then be an ally in discovering possible early symptoms and in weighing the advantages against the disadvantages of this treatment. In general, the physician should avoid authoritarian statements such as "While tardive dyskinesia is a risk, you need to take your medication" since this position will engender avoidance rather than compliance [31]. It might be better to say, "I don't want to see you needing to go back into the hospital all the time, and this medication will prevent that. If we follow your medication carefully, this side effect called tardive dyskinesia can be kept to a low risk." This warning cannot be used with patients who prefer hospitalization because they will use it as a reason to discontinue neuroleptics [32].

While the previous discussion contains many general issues, several specific issues of medication management need to be addressed: dosage, side effects, complications, family issues, transference, distortions, and countertransference.

Dosage

Most psychoactive medications have half-lives that approach or exceed 24 hours and, therefore, permit once-a-day dosages [33]. This can help reduce the noncompliance problems that frequently occur with multiple dosages. Patients need to know how long the medication is intended to last, or else they may conclude they are getting treated for four to eight hours only or perhaps just for sleep problems. These assumptions can quickly erode any belief that the medication could possibly help them.

In general, a useful goal is to increase the dose to therapeutic levels as rapidly as the patient's comfort and safety will permit. The patient should be informed of this objective and then invited to collaborate on it. This also means the patient should be informed of the most common adverse effects of the drug before medication is started. With this knowledge, the patient can make better decisions at home about when to increase the dosage of the medication. Rigid schedules frequently fail because they do not take the patient's psychological and physiological sensitivities into account. With more flexibility, the patient can be given small doses of the medication to be increased as comfort permits. Psychiatric medications are unusual compared with many other types of medications in that initial doses are often much lower than final doses. Physicians should tell patients this and give them an estimate of a desirable final dose range so they don't feel the starting dose has been arbitrarily increased four-fold or eight-fold. Some very regressed and/or dysfunctional patients cannot make these simple dosage decisions. In these situations, more frequent visits and phone contacts are necessary.

Prescribed dosage changes after symptom remission may have a variety of possible meanings to the patient, and the clinician should explore them with the patient before changing the dosage. Dose reduction schedules designed to lower long-term dosages may be interpreted as license to reduce to zero. Any reduction may imply to some patients that they are perfectly well and in no need of further assistance. On the other hand, reductions may be frightening to patients fearing relapse since the medication represents a stable protector. Increases in dosage may demoralize those who take this as a sign of an ever-worsening condition.

Certain dosage schedules for anxiety (or pain) can increase the risk of addiction to sedatives/hypnotics [34]. The more reinforcing the taking of medications, the greater the risk of addiction. This risk increases if the amount of distress is great, the relief from distress is rapid, and distress is heightened by withdrawal symptoms when the medication is stopped. Thus, the prescribing of a fast-acting, short-lived anxiolytic to be taken p.r.n. only when a patient becomes very anxious would maximize the risks of addiction. This patient would experience many episodes of rapid relief associated with pill taking. Once-a-day or scheduled, divided dosages with a longer acting anxiolytic that maintains relief between doses would help minimize the pairing of relief with pill taking and would eliminate many minor withdrawals.

Adverse Effects

Some of the most disturbing adverse effects, such as sedation with antidepressants and benzodiazepines, dystonias with neuroleptics, and nausea with lithium, are transient and tend to occur in the first week [33]. Patients who are informed that these side effects are temporary and who know what to do about them can tolerate them better and will be better treatment allies. Patients then should be encouraged to call their physicians regarding adverse effects that are disturbing and unexpected. Often, just having this option is enough to reassure patients to continue with medication.

Some patients may complain of symptoms that the physician does not believe are side effects. The physician must respond to these symptoms as well as explain to the patient why they are probably not side effects. The physician's continuing concern can be expressed by inquiring about the symptoms during future visits. In this climate, the patient can feel comfortable mentioning other symptoms that might be subtle side effects. For example, with neuroleptics, akathisia is the most common adverse effect leading to medication noncompliance [35]. Detection of mild forms of akathisia requires both skilled observation and a patient who feels that his/her symptoms are important to the physician.

It is not only important to define the adverse effects themselves, but also to explore the patient's reactions to them. Side effects can be interpreted in psychotic ways. For example, the patient may view dystonia, retrograde ejaculation, amenorrhea, and galactorrhea as control by others or as the product of malignant intent. Depressed patients might view their side effects as further punishment.

Side effect-prone patients Highly anxious patients, including agoraphobics [36], are also prone to report side effects, many of which are actually symptoms of anxiety [37]. Even on placebos, they complain of numerous side effects and are prone to discontinue the medication [38]. These patients will be hypervigilant for side effects and will exaggerate original symptoms they fear are side effects. They may complain of dizziness, tingling in the extremities, GI disturbance, headaches, palpitation, dry mouth, and other symptoms that accompany anxiety. Before starting these patients on medication, the physician should scrupulously review and record the presenting symptoms so the patient will understand what symptoms will probably not be considered adverse effects. Later, as side effects appear, the physician must clearly screen true drug-related ones. These patients generally tolerate medication better with ample reassurance and explanation. They should not be given a detailed list of possible side effects as there is a substantial risk of suggestion-induced effects [37].

Occasionally, a patient will present with a history of bizarre and bewildering side effects to homeopathic doses of medications. Sometimes a brief placebo trial is useful with such a patient so that such responses can be documented and later explained to the patient. If the physician conducts the placebo trial in a caring and understanding fashion, the patient will not feel as if he/she has been exposed. An anxious patient can be told that the anxiety is so severe his/her mind and body are producing these reactions to placebo. This explanation generally is experienced as acceptable and non-condemning. The following case demonstrates how a placebo trial can be used.

> *Case 3.* Mrs. S., a 29-year-old married woman with a three-year history of panic attacks progressing to general anxiety and later depression, was referred because she was "refractory to medication." She had multiple somatic complaints and listed numerous medications to which she was either "allergic" or had developed major side effects, sometimes "ruining my nervous system." She denied that significant marital conflict or numerous geographic moves were related to her anxiety. She said "I know that stress can make you feel nervous, but not like this. This is in my body. There is something wrong with my body." She had had myriad negative medical investigations for complaints such as dyspnea, dizziness, or tachycardia. A neurologist finally concluded that she had panic attacks and started

her on imipramine. She stated that during a seven-day trial of 50 mg of imipramine each day she felt "hyper," dizzy, and had tingling in her hands and palpitations. While these could have been adrenergic side effects, she had noted similar reactions to drugs that had no possibility of creating these side effects. She was angry at physicians "who made me go through these ordeals."

Because of these problems, she was hospitalized and started on trazodone 50 mg, but she refused to take more than one evening dose. She complained of dyspnea, tachycardia, insomnia, and feeling like her mind was racing all night. She insisted that these had to be drug effects and that her mind could never have created such a strong reaction. Because she said that the benzodiazepine, oxazepam, had helped her anxiety, but not her depression or her panic attacks, a trial of alprazolam, a potentially antidepressant benzodiazepine, was begun. Mrs. S. was reassured that alprazolam was very similar to oxazepam, the one medication she tolerated. In spite of this, she reported a reaction to 1 mg alprazolam h.s. nearly identical to one she had had to trazodone. Psychotherapy and even relaxation training remained stalled because of her insistence that there was a physical problem.

A placebo trial was then initiated. After placebo, she again complained of insomnia, racing thoughts, dyspnea, and dizziness. A one-hour session was then scheduled with her to go over the results of these trials. The patient was told we had evidence that her mind was more powerful at creating physical symptoms than we had suspected. The results of the placebo trial were then reviewed. She was told that her panic and anxiety disorder was indeed severe and that she may have developed a phobia of medications in general that exacerbated her symptoms when she took any pill. She agreed that this could be true because she remembered developing some symptoms just before and just as she was taking the medication. When Mrs. S. asked if this meant all her symptoms were just in her mind she was told that her mind was capable of producing these very real symptoms.

She then asked questions about how panic attacks could be psychological, and if we were recommending medication for them. The patient was told that everybody has a different threshold for developing a panic attack, that hers was probably low, and that this low threshold might be raised by the medication.

I explained to her that fear of abandonment or being left alone was a common stress that triggers panic attacks and that this fear develops from thoughts and feelings about specific events in her life. Mrs. S. then described having had panic attacks earlier in her life when she was going through a divorce and that this was a time during which she feared being alone. We talked about how psychotherapy dealing with this fear and with her catastrophizing might further help her. She agreed and then wanted to know if we would start medications again. She was told that this would be up to her and that she probably would still be phobic and have anxiety reactions to the drugs. She then insisted on a drug trial, preferring to start fresh with a drug to which she had not yet developed a phobia. Because of her covert, hostile, dependent style with physicians, a mildly skeptical approach was also used. Side effects would regularly be predicted, and expectation about positive effects would be scaled down.

A trial of phenelzine was started. This time the patient said she was aware of feeling more "hyper" after taking it but then realized that was probably due to her anxiety and not to the drug. She did relatively well on the drug, although she continued to seek nearly daily reassurance about mild, vague anxiety-related "side effects." She also began to engage in a cognitive-behavioral approach in individual psychotherapy and to examine conflict resolution in marital therapy. It appeared that the placebo trial had helped her to understand her reactions to drugs as well as to accept a more psychobiologically based model for her problems.

Family Influence

The family's attitude toward the treatment must be assessed and, if necessary, active interventions must be used to develop an alliance with them. On the simplest level, this means having the family come in, ask questions, and get an understandable explanation of the treatment. Family members will want to know on very concrete levels what to do with a patient, and they should be given direct, concrete answers if possible. The family, like the patient, needs an explanation that integrates the patient's experience with biological and psychological approaches to treatment. The clinician can use these meetings to explore and clarify the positive or negative biases family members frequently have about medication. This dovetails nicely with an

approach to family therapy for schizophrenics that has been shown
to lower relapse rates [39]. The family can learn to recognize the
patient's stresses and psychotic symptoms as well as how medications
can help (see Chapter 9).

Compliance is improved if a spouse or partner assumes a supervisory role [27]. This advantage must be balanced against the
patient's desire and capability for autonomy. It the patient is
attempting to adhere to a medication regimen, but is unsuccessful
because of cognitive or emotional disorganization, specific aids can
be considered. In many cases, use of a pill counter or depot fluphenazine and other approaches can help preserve the patient's autonomy
and minimize other family members' overinvolvement.

If a patient is noncompliant, incapable of autonomous functioning, and seriously in need of medication, significant others
(including employers or landlords) can be enlisted as allies [20]. The
therapist must then determine who will be the best ally. Frequently,
even in very pathological families, one family member has a good
relationship with the patient and appears genuinely concerned about
the patient's well-being. Asking the patient if such a person exists
is usually the most direct and accurate way of finding such an ally.
This person will need ample support from the physician because the
patient may continue to resist taking medication and other family
members may attempt to sabotage this new supervisory/therapeutic
arrangement. Goldhamer [40] suggests that in schizophrenic's
families with high expressed emotion, the family should not be
involved at all in supervising medications because their controlling
style will increase the risk of relapse.

Sometimes the best ally will not be a person who has the best
relationship with a patient but rather a person who has the most
leverage, such as a landlord or employer. It may be necessary to
make further employment or tenancy conditional on taking medication and receiving therapy. With this arrangement, the employer or
landlord who might have terminated the patient's employment or
tenancy may reconsider. Contact with any of these people needs to
be made with the patient's informed consent. Ideally, such contact
and meetings can be conducted with the patient present. If this is
not possible, the patient should be informed of all that transpired.
Legally, the therapists must have the patient's informed consent to
tell others about the patient, but he/she does not need this consent
to listen to others speaking about the patient. Therapeutically, trust
will best be maintained if the patient is told of any meetings with
others at which the therapist just listens.

If a family subverts the treatment because its members are invested in homeostasis and control and not in the patient's improvement, family therapy should be considered. Even when these problems are not present, family therapy is valuable in the treatment of acute schizophrenia (see Chapter 9). The following case demonstrates several issues regarding their medication compliance.

Case 4. Mr. H., a 33-year-old single man, was readmitted to the state hospital for an acute exacerbation of schizophrenia. He had had over ten hospitalizations in the previous six years and routinely stopped taking his medication upon discharge. During remissions, he functioned adequately. He had a girlfriend with whom he spent much time and a job as a mechanic at a rural garage. There were no family members in the immediate vicinity. Mr. H. had been treated with depot fluphenazine in the past, but invariably stopped coming to appointments to get his injections.

This time he was started on intramuscular fluphenazine again with the plan that he and his girlfriend would come in every two weeks to discuss how the couple had been doing. They both agreed to this plan, as each saw conflict areas in the relationship and felt they might benefit from counseling. For two months this plan worked well because it insured that he would come to get medication as well as to handle problems in his personal life. It also became clear that Mr. H.'s girlfriend liked to mother him and that she could not do this as he improved and stabilized. More conflict arose between the pair, resulting in his not wanting to come in to get his medication because he "did not need it anymore, no matter what J (girlfriend) or those doctors say." For him, not taking medications was an assertion of independence in their relationship, but also a way of ultimately reestablishing a more dependent relationship.

The therapists decided ongoing couple's therapy was needed and increased leverage would be necessary to get Mr. H. to take his medication. It was also decided that, if possible, his girlfriend shoud not assume a supervisory role because this would promote an already pathological dependency relationship in which the girlfriend was ambivalent about Mr. H. staying well.

A conference was then held with Mr. H.'s employer. He indicated that Mr. H. had been "a fairly good employee as long as he just worked on the cars and didn't deal with the customers too much." The employer was concerned about the annual or semiannual trips to the state hospital and had been thinking of laying the patient off. As a compromise, he agreed to give Mr. H. time off to get his medications and to make this a condition for continued employment. We told the employer this plan probably would reduce, but not necessarily eliminate, the need for hospitalization. He said he could probably tolerate the hospitalizations if they were no more frequent than every 18 months. He then asked several questions about Mr. H. such as "What should I do when he starts talking to the radio?" Further discussion revealed this was an early sign of relapse. The employer was encouraged to call one of the therapists if this occurred.

Subsequent to this meeting, Mr. H. enjoyed a long remission. He never completely accepted the need for continued medications, but liked the idea of adding oral fluphenazine to treat the early symptoms of acute exacerbation of his illness, such as insomnia and thought broadcasting. The couple's therapy went better as Mr. H. and his girlfriend adjusted to more equal roles in their relationship.

SYMBOLIC DISTORTION AND TRANSFERENCE

Patients can attribute a variety of latent meanings to pharmacotherapy. The physician can minimize the destructive effects of these interpretations if they are anticipated and explored as soon as possible. This objective can be accomplished by systematically investigating the meanings patients attach to receiving medications, to the drugs themselves, and to their effects. Unlike dynamic psychotherapy, these meanings need not be explored past the objectives of medication management.

Frequently, the act of prescribing medication has symbolic implications. Patients who view therapists prescribing medications as nurturing will have a more positive transference to the therapist if he/she prescribes medication. Similarly, if a request for medication is denied, then a patient may feel that the physician is withholding. While this distortion is frequently based on transference, it may also result from strong cultural beliefs.

In many cultures a physician should always prescribe something. Cultural values may be so strong that a continuing therapeutic relationship with the patient is contingent on prescribing some medication even though the physician believes that the patient does not need medication. Here the physician must find a balance between the narrower goal of optimal medical treatment (no medications) and the broader goal of the patient's improved well-being. Ideally, the patient can overcome this cultural belief, but in reality this may not be feasible. In such cases, homeopathic doses of medications might be considered. The following case demonstrates how this approach can be used.

> *Case 5.* Mrs. R., a 42-year-old married Hispanic woman, came to our crisis clinic because she had been feeling extremely anxious for about a week. She stated that a friend of hers had been severely battered eight days previously and after this, the patient became fearful that the same would happen to her. She indicated she had always been somewhat "high-strung, but nothing like this." Her complaints included poor concentration, startling easily, occasional palpitations, and insomnia. At the beginning of the interview, Mrs. R. had pressured speech, but by the end of the interview, she appeared calmer and seemed to be seeing her situation more realistically. Because of her good response to the supportive interview, several more were scheduled. She readily agreed and then asked what pills she would be getting. While I believed her acute anxiety would probably respond rapidly to a few more supportive therapy sessions, I assumed she would probably not accept this approach by itself. When continued therapy was discussed with her, she continued to ask for pills "for the days I can't see you." The placebo response rate for acute anxiety is approximately 80 percent [41]. I decided to give her diazepam 2 mg t.i.d. I selected diazepam because it had a long duration of effect if higher doses were required; I prescribed it three times a day to enhance the placebo effect. I told her this dose was too strong for some people and if this was true for her she could halve the pills. The patient was also told that she might not need the full week's supply. Before leaving, she was instructed to lower her coffee intake from six cups a day to two cups a day, to use decaffeinated coffee if she wished more than two cups, and to use decaffeinated coffee all the time if that was acceptable to her.
>
> She returned in four days as scheduled and stated that she felt better. She confessed that she had taken the medication mainly when she felt the need for it and said that just knowing it was there often helped her feel better. Mrs. R. reported that

she took approximately one to two tablets a day, noted that they were not too strong, and that on one occasion she took two to fall asleep. When the patient inquired about taking the tablets regularly so she wouldn't be "so high-strung," I discussed the risks and problems of long-term diazepam usage. She accepted the possibility that pills might help acute anxiety but not chronic anxiety. We reviewed various means of controlling anxiety, including biofeedback, relaxation training, meditation, exercise, and cognitive-behavioral therapy. Only biofeedback and relaxation training were acceptable to her. She was given referrals to follow up on these possibilities and was scheduled for one more supportive therapy session. No further prescriptions were needed.

Other patients will regard the prescribing of medications as evidence the physician is not interested in them as people. This too can be a result of transference and/or a strong cultural belief. In such cases, this belief needs to be explored and, if possible, medications should be delayed until the conflict is resolved. As therapeutic effects become evident, patients may then perceive medications as a threat. They may conclude that they do not have any personal control over their illnesses or see the clinician's prescribing medications as a narcissistic injury since chemicals could accomplish what they couldn't [42]. These feelings will also need to be anticipated.

Patients may also have symbolic distortions in regard to the medication itself. As Gutheil [42] noted, this frequently takes the form of personifying the medication and/or attributing magical meaning to the treatment regime. Forms of personification may include seeing the medication (with the physician's name always on the bottle) as a part of the physician or attributing human qualities to medications, with Stelazine® being a female named Stella and Haldol® a male named Hal. Thus, a male patient with homosexual fears might balk at taking Haldol, but have no resistance to taking Stelazine (unless he also believed that Stelazine would make him more female). The drug ritual regarding timing and amounts of dosages also may acquire magical or superstitious properties. All these distortions could make instituting or changing medications very difficult. The sensitive clinician needs to facilitate patients' communications about these beliefs.

Cost of medications may be a real or distorted reason for resistance to taking them. However, many patients are uncomfortable discussing these costs and will not initiate questions on the subject. In such cases, the physician should explain and inquire about costs. Some patients will be less resistant if they are prepared before they get the pharmacy bill. The physician can then help the patient view these costs within the large context of the illness. In most cases, the patient can eventually see that the expenses are small compared with the problems of his/her illness. Most patients like tips on how they can save money on their medication such as calling several pharmacies for prices. They may want to know if the physician had considered a generic drug to help cut costs or a different but related drug that was less expensive [43]. All this information can give patients more understanding or a sense of control when purchasing medication. It may also help correct a common distortion that physicians are wealthy and are insensitive to others' financial problems. Occasionally, financially secure patients may have opposite reactions to this information. They may feel the physician thinks they cannot afford the medication and thinks they are not good enough for a brand name prescription. However, overt questions are not necessary with these patients because they usually communicate their need to be seen as wealthy in many other ways.

Many patients are also uncomfortable discussing adverse effects related to sexual or bowel function. Patients who are paranoid, in particular, would never dare ask questions about sexual or bowel function because they might assume that the physician is trying to control these functions. The physician should initiate such discussions with questions such as, "Are the pills causing any constipation?" If the patient notices changes in sexual functioning, it will be important to ascertain if these are really side effects and, if so, how the patient understands and views them. Side effects are not always perceived negatively. Male obsessive-compulsive patients may like retrograde ejaculation because it is "cleaner."

COUNTERTRANSFERENCE AND SUPERSTITIONS

Psychopharmacotherapists are presented with unique opportunities to develop and act out countertransference. If they become too identified with the prescribing and efficacy of medications, problems usually ensue. For example, manics may need to fail by discontinuing lithium several times before they become convinced that lithium is important to use prophylactically. Physicians may go to great lengths and add unnecessary medications in the attempt to prevent an inevitable failure. The urge to write another prescription or to exercise more authority can become very great. Some patients who are diagnosed as having personality disorders may be placed on multiple medications or multiple elaborate trials of medications because they do not (or as sometimes viewed, will not) respond to medications. The pharmacotherapist, unwilling to accept that the medications do not work, then tries medications "just one more time." In these situations the physician must look at his/her own feelings of omnipotence rather than write more prescriptions.

Superstitious learning may occur if the physician tries a new medication or a novel use of a familiar medication and the patient coincidentally improves. The physician might then routinely begin using this new approach. Because the physician's zeal and interest in the new approach will augment the placebo response [12], many patients will appear to improve. Further patterns may emerge concerning responders and nonresponders, all of which could be based on chance. The end result can be an otherwise competent physician making such statements as "I have found in those psychotic, little, old ladies, that a little diazepam seems to improve their mood and their psychosis" or "I don't know why but valproate acid seems to work on some of these men with obsessive thoughts, so now I routinely use it on obsessives." These may be brilliant, creative, new endeavors, but in the absence of more controlled testing, they are more likely manifestations of the placebo effect with biased testing. Frequently, these same physicians eventually abandon last year's cures for this year's new one that "really seems to work."

For the physician to avoid this problem, he/she must stay highly sensitized to the power of the placebo effect. Thirty to forty percent of depressed or schizophrenic patients will respond significantly to placebo [33], and 80 percent [35] of acutely anxious patients will respond. All personal conclusions derived from clinical data with small samples are suspect unless double-blind placebo controls were used. More detailed ramifications of this distorted learning process are described elsewhere [44].

CONCLUSION

Skillful psychopharmacology requires sensitivity to the patient's experience and flexibility in approach. An understanding of patient compliance and the placebo effect are also important. Fortunately, most approaches recommended herein to enhance compliance have also been shown to enhance the placebo effect and vice versa. These approaches should be pursued to create a good working alliance with the patient and to help with his/her problems, but not to trick the patient. The psychopharmacologist must inform patients about their treatment and must routinely attempt to understand the patient's experience and to correct distortions and misconceptions. The best approach will be unique to each patient and should be derived from an empathic understanding of the patient and a broad working knowledge of psychopharmacology and psychotherapy.

REFERENCES

1. May ORA: Antipsychotic drugs and other forms of therapy. In *Psychopharmacology, a review of progress 1957-1967*, edited by Efron D H. Washington, DC: US Government Printing Office, 1967, pp. 1155-1176
2. Epstein PS, Fawcett J: Clinical Management-Imipramine-Placebo Administration Manual. NIMH Psychotherapy of Depression Collaborative Research Program: Pharmacotherapy Training Center, Rush Presbyterian St. Luke's Medical Center, Department of Psychiatry, 1980
3. Byrly H: Explaining and exploiting placebo effects. *Perspect Biol Med* 19: 423-436, 1976
4. Jospe M: *The Placebo Effect In Healing*. Lexington, Massachusetts: Lexington Books, D.C. Heath and Company, 1978
5. Chodoff P: Paternalism versus autonomy in medicine and psychiatry. *Psychiatr Ann* 13:318-320, 1983
6. Ackerman TF: Why doctors should intervene. *Hastings Center Report* 12: 14-17, 1982
7. Cross AW, Churchill LR: Ethical and cultural dimensions of informed consent. *Ann Intern Med* 96:110, 1982
8. Docherty JP, Marder SR, Van Kammen DP, Siris SG: Psychotherapy and pharmacotherapy: conceptual issues. *Am J Psychiatry* 134:529-533, 1977
9. Trux CB, Mitchell KM: Research on certain therapist interpersonal skills in relation to process and outcome. In *Handbook of Psychotherapy and Behavioral Change*, edited by Garfield SL, Bergin AE. New York: John Wiley and Sons, 1970, pp. 299-344
10. McGlashan TH: Intensive individual psychotherapy of schizophrenia. *Arch Gen Psychiatry* 40:909-920, 1983
11. Kahana RJ, Bibring GL: Personality types in medical management. In *Psychiatry of Medical Practice in a General Hospital*, edited by Zinberg N. New York: New York International University Press, 1964
12. Shapiro D: *Neurotic Styles*. New York: Basic Books, 1965
13. Carr JE: Differentiation similarity of patient and therapist and the outcome of psychotherapy. *J Abnorm Psychol* 76:361-369, 1970
14. *Diagnostic and Statistical Manual Disorders*, 3rd ed (DSM III). Washington DC: American Psychiatric Association, 1980
15. Yalom ID: *The Theory and Practice of Group Psychotherapy: The Help-Rejecting Complainer*. New York: Basic Books, 1975, pp. 399-404

16. Brody S: Syndrome of the treatment-rejecting patient. *Psychoanal Rev* 51: 75-84, 1964
17. Haley J: *Strategies of Psychotherapy.* New York: Grune and Stratton, 1963
18. Shapiro AK, Morris LA: The placebo effect in medical and psychological therapies. In *Handbook of Psychotherapy and Behavioral Change: An Empirical Analysis*, 2nd ed, edited by Garfield SL, Bergin AE. New York: John Wiley and Sons, 1978, pp. 369-410
19. Papp P: The Greek chorus and other techniques of paradoxical therapy. *Family Process* 19:45-57, 1980
20. Selvini MP, Boscolo L, Cecchin G, Prata G: Hypothesizing-circularity-neutrality: three guidelines for the conductor of the session. *Family Process* 19:3-12, 1980
21. Diamond RJ: Enhancing medication use in schizophrenic patients. *J Clin Psychiatry* 44:(6) section 2, 7-14, 1983
22. Levine P, Britten AF: Supervised patient management of haemophilia. *Ann Intern Med* 78:105-201, 1973
23. Rosenburg SG: Patient education leads to better care for heart patients. *HSMHA Health Reports* 86:793-802, 1971
24. Katon W: Doctor-patient negotiation and other social science strategies in patient care. In *The Relevance of Social Science for Medicine*, edited by Eisenburg L, Kleinman A. Dordrecht Holland: Reidel, 1981, pp. 253-279
25. Morris LA, Halperin JA: Effects of written drug information on patient knowledge and compliance: a literature review. *Am J Public Health* 69: 47-52, 1979
26. Ley P: Comprehension, memory and the success of communication with the patient. *J Inst Health Educ* 10:23-29, 1972
27. Blackwell B: Treatment adherence. *Br J Psychiatry* 129:513-531, 1976
28. Rudd P: In search of the gold standard for compliance measurement. *Arch Intern Med* 139:627, 1979
29. Prien R: Continuation therapy in depression: preliminary findings from a multi-hospital collaborative study. Presented at the American College of Neuropsychopharmacology Annual Meeting, San Juan, Puerto Rico, December 16-18, 1980
30. Herz MT, Melville C: Relapse in schizophrenia. *Am J Psychiatry* 137:801, 1980
31. Leventhal H, Singer R, Jones SH: The effects of fear and specificity of recommendation. *J Pers Soc Psychol* 2:20-29, 1965
32. Havens LL: Some difficulties in giving schizophrenia and borderline patients medication. *Psychiatry* 26:289-296, 1963
33. Klein DF, Gittelman R, Quitkin F, Rifkin A (eds): *Diagnosis and Drug Treatment of Psychiatric Disorders: Adults and Children*, 2nd ed. Baltimore: Williams and Wilkins, 1980
34. Carlin AS, Ward NG: Medication abuse and misuse in health care. In *Behavioral Science in the Practice of Medicine*, edited by Carr JE, Dengerink H. New York: Biomedical Publishing Unit/Elsevier Publishing Company, 1983
35. VanPutten T: Why do schizophrenic patients refuse to take their drugs? *Arch Gen Psychiatry* 31:67-72, 1974
36. Zitrin CM, Klein DF, Woerner MG: Treatment of agoraphobia with group exposure in vivo and imipramine. *Arch Gen Psychiatry* 37:63-72, 1980

37. Shapiro AK, Chassan J, Morris LA, Frick R: Placebo-induced side effects. *J Op Psychiatry* 6:43–46, 1974
38. Marks I: Are there anticompulsive or antiphobic drugs? Review of the evidence. *Psychopharmacol Bull* 18:78–84, 1982
39. Goldstein MJ, Rodnick EH, Evans JR, et al: Drug and family therapy in the aftercare of acute schizophrenics. *Arch Gen Psychiatry* 35:1169–1177, 1978
40. Goldhamer PL: Relapse in schizophrenia. *Arch Gen Psychiatry* 38:842–843, 1981
41. Rickels K: Predictors of response to benzodiazepines in anxious outpatients. In *The Benzodiazepines*, edited by Gavattini S, Mussini E, Randall LO. New York: Raven Press, 1972, pp. 257–281
42. Gutheil TG: The psychology of psychopharmacology. *Bull Menninger Clinic* 46:321–330, 1982
43. Weiner RD, Coffey CE, Campbell CP, Merritt MF: The price of psychotropic drugs: a neglected factor. *Hosp Comm Psychiatry* 34:531–535, 1983
44. Featherstone HJ, Beitman BD, Irby DM: Distorted learning from unusual medical anecdotes. *Med Educ* 18:155–158, 1984

CHAPTER 4

Introducing Medications During Psychotherapy

Bernard D. Beitman

Many variables influence the decision to introduce medications into psychotherapy. Most critical are the therapist's own biases for and against such treatment as discussed by Klerman (Chapter 2) and the diagnostic indications discussed by Weissman, Rush, Goldstein, Mavissakalian, and Eckert in the later chapters of this book. Other major influences include form of therapy (individual, group, family, marital), school of therapy (psychodynamic, cognitive, behavioral, existential), frequency and length of sessions, outcome criteria and goals (cost, symptom removal, prevention of relapse, interpersonal change), type of drug, route of administration, and treatment setting [1]. Also critical is whether or not treatment is to be split between a pharmacotherapist and a psychotherapist, as discussed by Chiles et al (Chapter 5).

In this chapter these complex variables are subordinated to the general task of predicting and hopefully controlling the influence of pharmacotherapy on the psychotherapeutic process. From this perspective, psychotherapy is perceived to be the primary treatment mode and pharmacotherapy is perceived to be a facilitator. In the previous chapter Ward reversed these priorities—psychotherapeutic concepts are utilized to maximize pharmacotherapeutic response.

In order to approach this task, individual psychotherapy must be defined in terms which respect differences but emphasize commonalities. This objective may be reached by recognizing that all forms and schools of psychotherapy involve relationships through time, and like the progression of the seasons, these relationships have stages with distinguishing characteristics [2]. In addition, pharmacotherapy must not be construed as some alien injection, totally separate and unlike the therapist's psychotherapeutic interventions. Instead, pharmacotherapy must be related to the context in which it is given by somehow conceptualizing it as part of the psychotherapeutic process. To highlight the importance of this requirement, it may be stated as follows:

Principle: When a medication is introduced into psychotherapy, it should be monitored and treated as if it resembled other therapeutic interventions.

One corollary may be added:

Corollary: The pharmacologic effects of any medication influence the psychotherapeutic process in both positive and negative ways. These effects may aid in the accomplishment of desired goals and may also prevent their attainment.

Previous attempts to describe the interaction between medications and psychotherapy have been generated primarily from a psychodynamic perspective. Great emphasis has been placed on the effect of medications upon the therapeutic alliance, upon the manner in which defenses may be altered, and the varieties of meaning which medications may assume for patients receiving them [3,7]. The last notion particularly continues to deserve explanation since medications may serve as powerful triggers for idiosyncratic thought-behavior-emotion complexes critical to therapeutic investigation.

The position taken in this chapter is a refinement of a previous attempt to lift the psychotherapeutic perspective on combined therapy out of the psychodynamic confines and place it in a broader context [8]. This integrating psychotherapy model is described in the following section. Subsequent sections describe the impact of medications introduced during each stage of the psychotherapeutic process.

A MODEL FOR INDIVIDUAL PSYCHOTHERAPY

The existence of many conflicting schools of psychotherapy challenges theorists and practitioners alike to define the common elements which allow each of these forms to be classified as psychotherapy. The model to be described is designed for individual psychotherapy, but is likely applicable to marital, family, and group approaches.

Individual psychotherapy is a series of events proceeding through time involving two people. Because it is a series of events through time, it may be called a process. Because it is a process, it may be arbitrarily divided into stages. (These stages can only approximate the reality of the relationship). Taken together, they may offer a map for the complex interpersonal terrain that is the psychotherapeutic relationship; they are, however, not the territory. Boundaries between stages may be difficult to delineate; elements of two or more stages may coexist at the same time. Stages may be traversed and subsequently reentered. Yet the stage concept provides a context from which to understand elements of the psychotherapeutic interaction. For example, a patient's focus on irrelevant matters or withdrawal from the therapist may suggest resistance during the early stages of therapy to the work of therapy, while each might indicate the patient's readiness to terminate during later stages.

The number of stages into which the process may be divided is arbitrary as are the labels given to them. This model (Table 1) entertains four stages with the potential for further subdivisions within each one. The term "engagement" is the label used for the first stage because it succinctly captures the primary purpose of the early part of treatment: for a person to accept the influence of another, he/she must trust and respect the other. The building of trust and respect results in psychological connection and commitment. Therapists may also require time in which to reach a committed position with each patient.

One marker of engagement is the patient's agreeing to follow the ground rules of therapy. The elements of the contract usually include fee, set length of sessions, and meeting time and place, and are usually accompanied by some attempts at role definition. Psychoanalysts, for example, encourage their patients to associate freely; cognitive-behavioral therapists encourage homework assignments, especially diaries; and existential therapists emphasize the value of here-and-now experiencing. These role definitions are designed to assist therapists in gathering information which may be useful in

Table 1. The Stages of Individual Psychotherapy

	Engagement	Pattern Search	Change	Termination
Goals	Trust Contract agreement Willing to be influenced	Define patterns to be changed	Transform maladaptive patterns into new thinking and behavior	Effect clean separation with maintenance of change
Methods	Empathic reception Specialized knowledge Offer of something which works Role definition	Silence Latent Content Questions Homework Instructions	Direct and indirect instructions to change thinking, feeling, and behavior patterns	Set termination date at at beginning, negotiate a date, or unilateral ending
Content	Presenting complaints Therapist-determined initial assessment content areas Role questions	Varies with therapist's theoretical positions—transference, cognitions, behavior, distant past, current relationship	Culturally approved adaptive patterns including self-reliance and responsibility as well as school specific lessons	Latent references to separation, review past losses, review gains of therapy, discuss future, appreciation
Resistance	Mistrust Contract disagreements Refusal to follow role expectations	Fear of self-confrontation	"Neurotic paradox"—desire to change without changing	Symptom recurrence, new problems
Transference	Distortions triggered by therapist appearance and by patient's previous therapy experiences	Reproduction of current and/or past relationships	Negative reaction to therapist's desire for change	Negative reactions to impending loss
Countertransference	Distortions triggered by patient's appearance and initial style	Evocation of therapist's relationships to others Experience of patient's internal states and/or style of interpersonal relationships	Negative reaction to patient's failure to change or to potential loss of patient through change	Negative reactions to separation

elucidating those patterns of thought-feeling-action which, if modified, would lead to satisfactory psychotherapeutic change. This objective is the primary purpose of the second stage which, therefore, is called "pattern search."

Therapies appear to differ most in both the manner in which information is sought and the ways in which this information is labelled and organized [2]. Common data-gathering includes listening to metaphorical communication (latent content), observing one's own emotional and fantasy response, organizing homework and out-of-the-office experiments, role playing in the office, observing transference, and paying attention to nonverbal communications. Therapists may remain silent, ask questions, give directions (including hypnosis), or nonverbally encourage patients to elaborate on the patterns requiring change. Although proponents of various schools may warn against the use of techniques from other schools, this warning must be held in abeyance until clearer evidence is available. Until then, therapists may consider all techniques at their disposal and attempt to solve the complex problem of selecting what technique should be used, in the hands of which therapist, working with what patient, at which time in therapy.

The way information is organized also appears to vary greatly among the schools. Psychoanalysts look for defenses against unconscious impulses and organize unconscious life according to sometimes clashing models of ego psychology, psychology of the self, and Kleinian approaches [9]. Cognitive-behavioral therapists [10] rely on the $A \rightarrow B \rightarrow C$ model, which is a simplified version of $S \rightarrow O \rightarrow R$. A (Activating event) triggers B (a Belief) and results in C (Consequence). Despite their complex models of unconscious functioning, psychoanalysts as well as most other therapists also use variants on $S \rightarrow O \rightarrow R$ (Stimulus) $\rightarrow O$ (Organism) $\rightarrow$ Response. For psychodynamic therapists it may be called the Rorschach principle: people bring to events their idiosyncratic interpretations which reflect basic underlying modes of organizing reality. The offer, ingestion, and effects of medications can serve, as do other stimuli, to evoke idiosyncratic reactions which reflect underlying psychological patterns.

The purpose of defining basic psychological patterns is to change them. Again, the schools of therapy appear to differ widely in regard to the content and form of their preferred methods. Despite many different terms and emphases, common factors seem to underly the efforts of therapists from widely differing persuasions [11-13]. Among these common change factors are suggestion, operant conditioning, emotional release, cognitive learning, and practice. The process of change appears divisible into three subsections, each with its own objective. First the identified pattern must be relinquished; the patient must decide that this thought-feeling-action complex must desist. Once maladaptive patterns are given up, they may be replaced by taking the often difficult first step in a new direction. Finally, to maintain the new pattern and hopefully generalize it to new situations, the patient must practice the new thought-feeling-action complex and work it through the old impediments and inertia [14].

As the new patterns become fixed in the patient's life, therapy becomes less necesary and termination ideally follows. The elements of the termination process are relatively predictable when contrasted with the wide range of possibilities inherent in the pattern search and change stages. Patients (and therapists) often have difficulty saying goodbye since one or the other may wish to prolong the relationship. New symptoms or old ones may appear, thus prompting the need to ignore the separation. Many other ploys and responses are potentially a part of this often difficult process. On the other hand, termination, like engagement, sometimes may be smooth and clean.

Each stage may be organized according to a general scheme. Each has a major goal, a discrete set of methods by which to reach that goal, characteristic content and likely interpersonal distortions, including resistance to the objectives of the stage, and stage-related transference and countertransference. For example, interpersonal distortions of the engagement stage are characterized by each participant's reactions to the surface appearance and manner of the other (e.g., age, sex, accent, race, socioeconomic class). During the second stage, each tends to react to more intimate details perceived in the other person's personality (seductiveness, passivity, pathological narcissism).

How does this stage model relate to pharmacotherapy? Generally speaking, the introduction of medications during any stage of therapy may serve as a method by which to gain the objective of the stage, a way to impede the reaching of those goals, and a trigger or symbol of interpersonal distortion. These points are illustrated in the following sections. But first, when does psychological management of pharmacotherapy become psychotherapy combined with pharmacotherapy?

WHEN DOES PHARMACOTHERAPY
BECOME PSYCHOTHERAPY?

In the previous chapter, Ward has outlined the use of psychotherapeutic concepts in the management of patients being treated with medications. From this perspective, no attempts are made to change the patient through psychological techniques; rather, psychotherapeutic understanding is used in the service of gaining patient cooperation with the medication regimen and in maximizing the placebo response. In clinical practice, this perspective is not easily held since patients in pharmacotherapy often attempt to introduce psychotherapeutic issues. Whether or not these issues are developed any further depends upon two variables: the pharmacotherapist's willingness to enter into psychotherapeutic exploration and the amount of time allotted for discussion of medication management.

In controlled studies of combined treatment, pharmacotherapists are generally instructed to limit their interactions to drug specific issues, but since patients often attempt to involve therapists in other issues, in clinical practice the therapist's interest is a critical factor. Time and frequency of meetings is the other controlling variable. If, during maintenance drug therapy, patient and therapist meet for 15 minutes once a month, discussion of desired effects, dosage, side-effects, and the writing of the prescription are likely to fill the time. However, if they meet for 30 minutes per month, then approximately 15 minutes may be left to discuss other matters. These "other matters" are likely to become psychotherapeutic issues. Depending upon the complexity of the drug management problems, meetings which take more than 30 minutes per month during the maintenance phase of drug therapy have a high probability of spilling over into psychotherapeutic investigation. For the purpose of the following discussion I define psychotherapy with medications as those professional relationships in which a patient taking medication meets with a pharmacotherapist more than 30 minutes per month.

ENGAGEMENT

During controlled studies of combined therapy, researchers generally administer drug or placebo at the outset of psychotherapy. Therefore, the influence of introducing medications during the latter stages of therapy has not been studied in these protocols. Since the purpose of the first stage is to develop trust in the therapist and belief in his/her competence [15], medications may help or hinder the accomplishments of these goals. For depression, some therapists advocate a two-stage model by which the patient is offered a medication trial which, if successful, may obviate the need for psychotherapy [16]. The increased energy and improved mood may propel the patient out of the negative spiral of hopelessness and despair, replacing it with a more positively reinforcing loop. If the medication trial is only partially successful, then the patient may be invited to embark on a course of psychotherapy, assuming another antidepressant is not to be considered. There are many other alternatives to the simple two-stage model. Medications and psychotherapy are also often offered simultaneously. As suggested by the discussion in the previous section, the difference between the two-stage model and the simultaneous model may be obscured during the medication management in the acute phase.

These alternatives remain possible for other medication as well. Low-dose neuroleptics may suffice without psychotherapy in some borderline patients; lithium alone is often quite sufficient with bipolar disease; imipramine and other anti-panic medications may suffice for panic and agoraphobia. Whether or not psychotherapy is included depends upon the predispositions of the psychiatrist and the patient.

Successful medication administration is a powerful engagement method, and many psychiatrists appear to use this technique.

Case 1. A 38-year-old woman presented with racing thoughts, auditory hallucinations, and delusions of persecution. A trial of perphenazine successfully quieted her anxieties and put distance between herself and her delusions. She viewed my handling of her psychosis to be compassionate as well. For administrative reasons, I referred her to another psychiatrist with whom she reached a stalemated, eroticized relationship from which the therapist uncomfortably fled by referring the patient to his wife's therapy group. Sensing the manipulation, the patient called me and requested reacceptance into treatment by stating "You helped me once and now I'd like you to help me again." Although she resumed the relationship with intense erotic fantasies, she persevered with the knowledge that she had been helped once before by this same person. Medication management had instilled hope for improvement, one of the common underlying factors of most psychotherapies [12].

Medications do not have to be pharmacologically successful to engage patients in therapy. The fact that they are offered in a caring, purposeful way and that they may provide a vehicle for useful interchange makes the placebo effect a powerful engagement tool as well.

Case 2. A 36-year-old single man sought help for his self-diagnosed manic-depressive illness. He had been treated with amitriptyline with great success, but he experienced times of hyperexcitability, irritability, and rages while taking that medication. He had decided that lithium was the best treatment for him. As he described his symptoms and his lifestyle, it quickly became clear that he was terribly isolated and very paranoid; these characteristics seemed independent of his apparent mood swings. Police were always after him, the landlord was constantly plotting to evict him, and store clerks consistently mistreated him. For 18 months lithium therapy remained the focus of treatment with occasional forays into investigations of his paranoid thinking. His descriptions of the drug effects followed by his lectures on the problems with the current economic system, and on politics and history dominated our interactions. People in the next room could hear him raging. Gradually we discovered that lithium offered very little help for him despite his history of mood swings and his father's positive reaction to lithium treatment for a more classic manic-depressive illness. By that time he had begun to allow me to express my opinions about him, and he began to confront the boredom and loneliness of his life. Medication management had provided a vehicle through which he could begin to trust me enough to listen to me and to express the feelings underlying his paranoid and isolated existence.

Medications are two-edged swords in the engagement stage since their adverse effects may hamper the attainment of trust in the therapist and belief in his/her competence.

Case 3. A 30-year-old woman with advanced Hodgkins disease and a demanding, highly critical, antagonistic personality style was begun on doxepin for depression before she had been engaged in a psychotherapeutic relationship. She gained little effect at 200 mg, and with some encouragement by her, the psychiatrist raised it to 300 mg. She suffered a grand mal seizure which offered a clear-cut reason to drop yet another in a long line of caregivers.

Paranoid patients are particularly vulnerable to misinterpreting side effects. Akathisia, dystonias, parkinsonian symptoms may easily be interpreted as therapist malevolence.

Case 4. One 24-year-old paranoid schizophrenic asked to be treated with doxepin because he was depressed and because 80 mg of thiothixene was no longer helpful. However, after a two-month trial, he reported he did not like the side effects, which appeared minimal by his description. The medication seemed to be helping his sleep and perhaps alleviating his depression. The therapist, therefore, decided to encourage him to take it. Instead he hid the pills from three subsequent prescriptions and killed himself with an overdose, apparently fearing among other things that the therapist was trying to harm him.

Distortions

Patients and therapists respond to the idea of medications in a variety of distorted ways. Patients may perceive the medication offer to be a distancing maneuver through which the therapist is demonstrating a desire not to be engaged in a personal relationship. On the other hand, some patients find the offer of medications essential, especially if they perceive the therapist to be withholding in other ways (eg, silence, passivity). This spectrum of responses may be classified as transference reactions since it reflects intrinsic, idiosyncratic patterns of perceiving the actions of another.

Case 5. A 28-year-old narcissistic woman presented with daily migraine headaches and episodic anxiety. She had a history of physician-prescribed codeine abuse. Because her anxiety was often incapacitating, she requested diazepam. She was also clearly testing my ability to trust her with this request and thereby attempting to gauge her willingness to trust me. Her relationships with most men were characterized by finding herself always deprecated and used by them as she had been deprecated by her father. When, early in treatment, I gave her a small number of 1 mg of diazepam, she idealized me as a perfect therapist for her. This response required careful monitoring during the remainder of a successful psychotherapy.

Therapists also may respond to medications in a range of distorted ways. Klerman (Chapter 2) has listed some of these as ideological conflicts. Therapists may see the medication as an indicator of reduced therapist power and tend to withdraw from the therapeutic interaction. This reaction appears most likely with the introduction of lithium carbonate since the medication is so effective in many bipolar patients. Nevertheless, Jamison and Goodwin [17] reported a survey in which twice as many patients as psychiatrists believed that psychotherapy was helpful in the treatment of manic-depressive illness. Some therapists believe that medications reduce patient motivation for therapy or interfere with the development of the transference. These are subjects of continuing debate, yet some evidence and much clinical experience do not suggest that medications reduce the motivation for therapy [18]; in fact, medication may increase motivation. The question of interference with the transference is one of the major points of the next section on pattern search: medications may highlight transference reactions by permitting therapists a different view into the patient's tendency to distort the behavior and intentions of others.

Psychiatrists may introduce medications into psychotherapy in ways which reflect their own negative or positive distortions of the patient. These distorted responses may therefore be termed symptoms of countertransference.

Case 6. During the engagement stage with a particularly troublesome 25-year-old unmarried man, a psychiatrist became frustrated with the patient's demands for medication and excessive reports of shifting side effects that seemed to accompany any medication use. In desperation she tried the patient on a monoamine oxidase inhibitor (MAOI) and left town for two weeks without clarifying the foods to be avoided and the person designated to be her back-up. These omissions appeared to be the product of unconscious anger at a noncooperative patient. The patient quit therapy soon thereafter.

Transference and countertransference reactions may spiral together to reach a stalemate which, in hindsight, began early in therapy. Medications may provide a matrix through which stalemate spirals are developed.

Case 7. A 28-year-old borderline woman, who presented herself for treatment in a very helpless, lost, and needy way, pleaded for antidepressants and antianxiety medications during the first interview. She had a history of suicide attempts, one almost fatal. There was no indication for the antianxiety medication yet I responded with the prescription-rescue response she seemed to wish to elicit [19]. She used her helplessness in many other circumstances (eg, her chair was too uncomfortable) to weave me into a web so tight that only a moderate overdose attempt followed by a hospitalization could break our relationship. I was relieved when she told me she had found a new therapist; the patient acknowledged my relief as she said goodbye.

PATTERN SEARCH

The purpose of the second stage is to define patterns of thought-feeling-actions which, if changed, would bring psychological benefit. It is marked in part by a great increase in the patient's willingness to explore those issues which are central to the presenting difficulties. This willingness is a product of the patient's engagement into the psychotherapeutic relationship. Not uncommonly, patients must first be engaged before they will accept medications.

Case 8. A 26-year-old paranoid graduate student, only two years in the United States after living all her life in Hong Kong, sought psychiatric help because of anxiety and isolation. When the therapist suggested a neuroleptic for her obvious psychotic thinking, the patient balked and came irregularly to apointments. She indirectly referred to fears of trusting the therapist and finally was lost to follow-up.

Once into the pattern search with patients not receiving medications, therapists may find themselves wondering whether or not to introduce them, especially when therapy seems to be stalemated. This silent question may lead to obsessions about the relative severity of biological symptoms, ruminations about whether to seek consultation, doubts about psychotherapeutic potency, and fears of what colleagues might say. In the following example, the psychiatrist went through many of these thoughts and introduced the idea to his patient with positive results.

Case 9. A 26-year-old borderline woman sought psychoanalytic psychotherapy because of difficulties in maintaining relationships with men. As she deepened her attachment to her therapist and converted her vengeful fantasies about her mother (tying her and cutting her breasts), she showed signs and symptoms of depression. Her therapist was very reluctant to offer medications and ruminated about the decision for weeks. Finally, he mentioned his belief that antidepressant therapy was worthwhile. She responded that she had been asking friends about antidepressants all week and welcomed the opportunity. This reply confirmed his intervention. Months later, after a positive medication response, they discontinued it. A few months later, she showed more moderate signs of depression, but they both agreed that they should wait to see if the symptoms abated. They did. (Contributed by David Joseph, MD)

Introduction of Lithium

Of the major psychiatric medications, perhaps lithium is most dramatic in its effects. Antidepressants may give people energy and neuroleptics may organize thinking, but many patients with positive responses to lithium report feeling as if their personalities have changed. And perhaps they have. They are no longer euphoric, filled with great new ideas and energy; they feel stable, "centered," organized, level. Their sexual drives, business lusts, grandiosity, and entertainment value are all reduced. No longer can they hide in depressions. These and other responses may be readily predicted when lithium is introduced into psychotherapy and, consequently, form an often neglected set of patterns worthy of psychotherapeutic consideration [17].

Jamison and Goodwin [17] have organized these patterns under the following categories:

1. *Realistic losses.* For many, the manic state may be described as an endogenous stimulant addiction intermittently reinforced by increased energy, decreased need for sleep, increased sexuality, and productivity without the guilt often engendered by the term "drug addict." It is a pristine state of ignorance that is lost with the diagnosis and treatment. It is replaced by negative social sequellae that include discrimination by some employers and social contacts because of "mental illness" and self-labelling as "defective." In addition, the decrease in thought speed leads to a sense of memory loss and of decreased intellectual capacity. Lithium-induced weight gain may be particularly troublesome for some. If tremors are not controllable, then work options are reduced, and, occasionally, tremulous patients are required to be yet more dependent upon others to help them with minor tasks.

2. *Symbolic losses.* Manic patients taking lithium may experience an increase in vulnerability due to the loss of perceived omnipotence and independence. Said one patient, "I thought everyone else was going half speed; now I realize I was going twice as fast. I do not like this adjustment to everyone else's pace. I want to feel in control the way I felt before." Lithium may become the symbol of these losses and may be angrily rejected because of this meaning.

3. *Unrealistic losses.* Lithium and psychotherapy may also come to represent the patient's failures resulting from both manic-poor judgment and other thwarted life ambitions.

4. *General issues.*

a. Denial of the bipolar illness, especially its severity and nature, is not uncommon. Denial may be fueled by the enjoyment of the mania, amnesia secondary perhaps to the real biochemical features of the illness (state dependent learning), and inability to recall the sheer volume of perceptions, cognitions and emotions.

b. Fear of recurrence often plagues patients who do permit themselves to face the meaning and difficulties inherent in mania and severe depression. They may go too far in the other direction by becoming unduly self-protective, monitoring their emotions very carefully, observing their sleeping and appetite changes with unnecessary persistence. They may, therefore, become quite self-involved and shut themselves away from others.

c. Whether bipolar patients taking lithium are excessively self-observant or not, they may become confused about the source of their moods. Is a moderate depression caused by a failure of lithium treatment, perhaps requiring an increased lithium blood level, or is the moderate depression secondary to interpersonal factors? Is it both biological and psychosocial and, if so, in what proportion? These questions are often very difficult to answer.

Case 10. A 45-year-old narcissistic woman taking lithium for her bipolar illness developed a strong positive attachment to her therapist which became the subject for transference interpretation. After a few months of fairly level functioning, she and her psychiatrist decided to lengthen the time between sessions. Around the same time, she was rejected by a former lover and asked her current lover to move out of her house. Two days after the decision to lengthen the time between meetings with her psychiatrist, she entered a moderate depression. Was it a bipolar breakthrough, loneliness, or hypothyroidism—since women over 40 appear to be at greater risk for developing hypothyroidism secondary to lithium prophylaxis [20]? The question required examination at both the medical and psychological levels.

Accurate discrimination between medication effects and psychological effects may be problematical for other medications beside lithium as well. Psychiatrists may have been able to conclude that anorgasmia in women taking MAOIs was probably psychological until recent reports that suggest anorgasmia is not an uncommon side effect of the medication itself [21].

d. Developmental tasks may be unchallenged or delayed as might also happen with drug addiction. The mania permits the patient to avoid having to confront the realities of separation and loss characteristic of each developmental phase.

Case 11. A 30-year-old man with onset of mania at age 18 continued to live in a world of artistic fantasy supported by his father's money and charged by his manic dreams. He was started on lithium at age 27, but stopped at age 29 to continue to enjoy the possibilities his manic euphoria promised him, to avoid commitment to his own more mundane potential, and to continue his dependence upon his father.

e. Family and genetic concerns are often of paramount concern. Parents worry that their children might inherit the disorder and children may want parents to acknowledge their own need for treatment. Children may overidentify with their parents and avoid separating themselves. Many patients feel guilty for the pain they have caused their family members as a result of their illness and do not know how to rectify it.

Pattern Search Distortions

In the same way that patients may resist exploring certain ideas, they may resist exploring medications as a useful adjunct to psychotherapy. Rather than attempt to cajole, order, or threaten a patient who fails to follow a given therapeutic expectation (eg, remains silent, obsesses about irrelevant material, fails to do homework assignment), psychodynamic therapists attempt to uncover the motivators for the refusal. Resistance to medications may also hide critical underpinnings of the presenting psychological difficulties.

Case 12. A 48-year-old married man, father of three, refused to take lithium despite the clear indications. Analysis of this resistance revealed that he was afraid to recover from his recurrent depressions because he would then be required to return to his job as an electrical engineer. Since he was on disability from his employer, he would be ineligible for further compensation when he resumed working. Should he become incapacitated with depression again, he would not receive more disability payments but would be retired early. He was afraid of early retirement. Further analysis of this sequence suggested he was more afraid of divorce than early retirement. His depression allowed him to avoid confronting his marriage. Eventually he and his wife did divorce. After the divorce, indications for lithium were not evident.

Requests for medications may signal transference distortions.

Case 13. A 47-year-old woman sought therapy for recurrent depressive episodes. Because of a suggestion of family history of affective disorder and the cyclic nature of her problem, she began a trial of lithium. At moderate doses she reported some relief but experienced side effects which greatly disrupted her life. She stopped taking the drug. As psychotherapy deepened into the pattern search, she asked for sleeping medications. She refused to elaborate on her symptoms of insomnia, but rather became more insistent that she receive sleeping medications. The demands escalated, and we approached a stalemate. Slowly she revealed that she was unable to go to sleep because she had sexual fantasies about me. She believed she needed the medication to help her overcome these thoughts. Therapy proceeded for two years, during which time a strong eroticized transference became a fixed part of our relationship. She would never permit discussion of her feelings toward me, but rather talked about other subjects or insisted, cajoled, and otherwise attempted to seduce me. Finally, after three unsuccessful terminations, she agreed that transfer to a woman therapist would hold more promise for her.

Therapists may focus on medications when they wish to avoid experiencing emotions triggered by their patients. For example, a psychiatrist offered diazepam to his attractive female patient who did not want or need it. Apparently he insisted because she had developed a strongly sexualized attachment to him which he found pleasing but wished to deny. The medication seemed more intended to calm him down [22].

Therapists may also fail to withdraw medication because of their own distorted reactions to their patients.

Case 14. A 26-year-old borderline woman was started on dexedrine and desipramine for her attention deficit disorder. The psychiatrist reasoned that he would withdraw the dexedrine after the desipramine began to work. The decision to offer the medication was difficult to make because the patient had a history of drug abuse and had attempted a number of suicides. Her school work improved on the regimen, but when she experienced some interpersonal failures, she began abusing the dexedrine. The therapist was caught unconsciously in a highly sexualized bond with her and could not bring himself to stop the dexedrine although they had agreed that he would if she abused the drug. The patient settled his dilemma by suggesting that her previous physician, who had prescribed many of her drugs of abuse, might also prescribe these. The psychiatrist took this way out. Unfortunately, this approach did not resolve the obvious countertransference blindness. Eventually she asked him to sleep with her. His refusal led to a series of events culminating in her suicide with an overdose of desipramine.

The treatment of bipolar illness with lithium carries with it a number of predictable countertransference problems [17]. Therapists may feel guilty about depriving their manic patients of their special state of being and collude with them to discontinue lithium. The loss of the hypomania may be a loss for the therapist as well, especially if he/she enjoyed the patient in this state.

Psychotherapy with bipolar patients taking lithium may induce frustration, anger, or helplessness in therapists. Lithium treatment notwithstanding, bipolar patients may show fluctuations in mood which reflect inconsistencies in their attitudes toward themselves, toward others, toward therapy, and toward lithium. Psychotherapists may therefore find it difficult to focus on previously agreed upon psychological problems and partial solutions because patients are operating from shifting mental/biochemical states. The cause of wide mood swings may often be difficult to define, and, therefore, patients may tend to blame the therapist. Therapists may react defensively to these accusations. In their manic or depressed phases, bipolar patients are often sensitive to indicators of rejection and may withdraw further from treatment, creating a feedback loop in a negative direction. The spiral may end with the therapist's sense of impotence, the patient's stopping lithium, and the necessity of hospitalization.

CHANGE

The process of change may be subdivided into three parts: relinquishing of the old pattern(s), initiation of new pattern(s), and maintenance and generalization through practice of the changes. Medications may play a part in each of these three subgoals of the process of change.

The giving up of old patterns may be linked to loosening of denial of medication responsive disorders.

Case 15. A 45-year-old narcissistic woman was repeatedly perplexed by her pattern of repeated rejections from intimate relationships with men. During one dramatic session she was able to assimilate the real possibility that she actually engineered these rejections. The realization was so startling to her that she experienced a flu-like syndrome without fever as she allowed herself to see her influence over others. After disavowing the patterns, she attempted to eliminate her fear of intimacy. However, she experienced a long hypomanic episode followed by a severe depression. She was more able to admit that she had previous mood swings of this severity and that possibly she was manic-depressive. She had not been able to accept the potential for this disorder until she had attempted to relinquish her interpersonal pattern.

Medications may aid in the initiation of change. Patients may be fully aware of the patterns requiring change but may be too depressed to carry out the new patterns. Mandell [23] described a young woman who became increasingly apathetic in response to apparently accurate transference interpretations. The patient was given an MAOI which helped increase her assertiveness and activity level, thereby creating a feedback loop that allowed her to practice and maintain changes.

Phobic patients may be helped to face fears by taking benzodiazepines. Marks [24] has described their use with simple phobics and Mavissakalian [25] has reviewed the literature on agoraphobia. Once the patient has decided to try to change, the antianxiety medication may make exposure smoother and quicker.

Working Through and the Maintenance of Change

Once a new way of thinking, acting, and feeling has been initiated, some patients are able to leave therapy without return to earlier symptoms and problems. For those who continue in therapy, the task is to work through new insights and behavior changes to maintain and generalize the initial therapeutic successes. As the following vignette suggests, pharmacotherapy can aid in the process of maintaining change.

> *Case 16.* A 32-year-old married woman with two children finally accepted that her husband's affairs during their ten years of marriage were not going to end. She had known about them for most of their married life but chose to ignore them and hoped they would stop. Confronting him about them only led to his becoming more secretive, but she still found evidence that they continued. She was deeply depressed about the situation, but was afraid to leave the marriage. Firmly intent upon conquering the problem through psychological means, she refused to consider any medications for her depression. Finally she decided to divorce her husband; he accepted. She resumed her career in dramatic fashion, started to become quite successful, and discontinued therapy. However, she found herself sinking back into her old depressions, which she understood very well but could not shake. She made a mild suicide attempt and returned to therapy open to the idea of antidepressants. She had the clear vegetative signs of early morning awakening, reduced appetite, and weight loss. Her response to desipramine was positive. With her newfound energy and confidence, she said she was able to put into effect what she had learned about herself and her relationships. After four months she discontinued psychotherapy; after 12 months she discontinued the desipramine.

Distortions

Patients and therapists may use medications to subvert the change process. Patients may discontinue medications when change is possible, and therapists may offer medication-responsive diagnoses in an effort to prevent their patients from changing. Because the indications for medications may sometimes be fuzzy, clinical judgment is more likely to be confounded by countertransference and transference distortions, especially if either participant has some reluctance about change.

TERMINATION

Change precedes termination. In the same way that either of the pair may be unwilling to change, they may also react negatively to the idea of termination. The offer of medications at the end of psychotherapy should be examined first for transference and countertransference distortions. As in any stage of treatment, it is always possible for the therapist to suddenly discover that the patient did indeed have a medication-responsive disorder or required a medication different from the one being prescribed. However, this possibility is increasingly unlikely as patients near the termination stage.

One of the more common patient reactions to any termination is to experience a reappearance of the presenting symptoms. Not uncommonly these symptoms are short-lived. However, they are often an expression of fear of loss of the therapist and consequent fear of loss of the therapeutic gains. If a therapist feels guilty about this regression, medications may be offered as a way to hold onto the patient, a way to subvert the termination process and to continue contact through medication.

Terminations which are forced by external circumstances may trigger distorted responses in either person which may manifest themselves around medications.

> *Case 17.* A 30-year-old psychiatric resident had been seeing an intermittently psychotic 32-year-old man for 18 months one to two times per week. The therapist was heavily invested in the patient who had made but modest gains. As the forced termination caused by his leaving the residency loomed only a few months away, the patient began to express his sadness and anger at the desertion. The therapist felt increasingly guilty and decided that he should consider starting the patient on lithium. Medications appeared to be the way to continue the symbolic contact after they separated and a low possibility chance at "cure."

This last case points toward the dilemma created by termination of a patient on medication. The patient has three choices if the therapist is leaving town: seek a medication manager, stop the medication, or find a pharmacotherapist who is also a psychotherapist. If the therapist does not leave town, can he continue only as medication manager? They can shorten the time, but they will resume talking about psychotherapeutic issues eventually. In a few cases of mine, the patients terminated on medications and gradually stopped them on their own.

SUMMARY AND CONCLUSIONS

When introducing pharmacotherapy into psychotherapy, psychiatrists should treat the intervention as similar to other psychotherapeutic activities. Pharmacotherapy can aid (and inhibit) the engagement process by demonstrating therapist competence (or incompetence). Patients may misread the offer, prescription, and/or ingestion of medications in ways which characterize their responses to other ambiguous interpersonal transactions. These responses may aid therapists in developing further understanding of their patients if these responses are examined and included in the evaluation process.

The introduction of lithium carbonate heralds a number of potential patterns worthy of psychotherapeutic examination including real and imagined losses, family concerns, and problems in defining bipolar versus "normal" mood variations. Finally, not only do patients react to pharmacotherapy with therapeutically critical distortions, but therapists too may use medications as a countertransference distortion as well.

Medications may aid the process of change, and their use during termination may reflect problems both participants have separating from each other.

Medications and psychotherapy ultimately have some actions in common; each has some influence on brain activity. The mechanisms are quite different at first glance. Psychotherapy influences the brain through sight and sound within the context of the therapeutic relationship, while medications generally operate through the mouth and bloodstream within the context of the pharmacotherapeutic relationship. Yet, as described by Rush in Chapter 7, medications and cognitive therapy appear equally effective in the treatment of depression. This suggests that some final common pathways is reached through these widely divergent approaches to brain function. The chemical attempt to bridge the gap between mind and brain foreshadows the theoretical attempt. Where in the brain and how do pharmacotherapy and psychotherapy converge?

ACKNOWLEDGMENT

The author thanks Paula A. Levine for her assistance.

REFERENCES

1. Karasu TB: Psychotherapy and pharmacotherapy: toward an integrative model. *Am J Psychiatry* 139:1102-1114, 1982
2. Beitman BD: Comparing psychotherapies by the stages of the process. *J Operational Psychiatry* 14:20-27, 1983
3. Ostow M (ed): *The Psychodynamic Approach to Drug Therapy.* New York: The Psychoanalytic Research and Development Fund, 1979
4. Lesse S: *Anxiety: Its Components, Development and Treatment.* New York: Grune and Stratton, 1970
5. Sarwer-Foner GJ: An overview of combined psychopharmacology and psychotherapy. In *Psychopharmacology and Psychotherapy*, edited by Greenhill MH, Gralnick A. New York: Free Press, 1983
6. Gutheil TG: Drug therapy: alliance and compliance. *Psychosomatics* 19: 219-225, 1978
7. Goldhamer PM: Psychotherapy and pharmacotherapy: the challenge of integration. *Can J Psychiatry* 28:173-177, 1983
8. Beitman BD: Pharmacotherapy as an intervention during the stages of psychotherapy. *Am J Psychotherapy* 25:206-214, 1981
9. Chessick RD: Current issues in intensive psychotherapy. *Am J Psychotherapy* 36:438-448, 1982
10. Beck AT, Rush AJ, Shaw BJ, et al: Cognitive therapy of depression. New York: Guilford Press, 1979
11. Marmor J: Common operational factors in diverse approaches to behavior change. In *What Makes Behavior Change Possible*, edited by Burton A. New York: Brunner/Mazel, 1976
12. Frank J: Restoration of morale and behavior change. In *What Makes Behavior Change Possible*, edited by Burton A. New York: Brunner/Mazel, 1976
13. Strupp HH: Psychoanalysis, "focal therapy" and the nature of the therapeutic influence. *Arch Gen Psychiatry* 32:127-135, 1975
14. Pentony P: *Models of Influence in Psychotherapy.* New York: Free Press, 1981
15. Strong SR: Social psychological approach to psychotherapy research. In *Handbook of Psychotherapy and Behavior Change*, edited by Garfield SL, Bergin AE. New York: John Wiley, 1978

16. Klerman G: Combining drugs and psychotherapy in the treatment of depression. In *Depression: Biology, Psychodynamics and Treatment*, edited by Cole J, Schatzberg A, Frazier S. New York: Plenum Press, 1976
17. Jamison KR, Goodwin FK: Psychotherapeutic treatment of manic-depressive patients on lithium. In *Psychopharmacology and Psychotherapy*, edited by Greenhill MH, Gralnick A. New York: Free Press, 1983
18. Rounsaville BJ, Klerman GL, Weissman MM: Do psychotherapy and pharmacotherapy of depression conflict? *Arch Gen Psychiatry* 38:24–29, 1981
19. Epstein L, Feiner AH: Countertransference. New York: Jason Aronson, 1979
20. Transbol I, Christiansen C, Baastrup PC: Endocrine effects of lithium I. Hypothyroidism, its prevalence in long term treated patients. *Acta Endocrinol* 87:759–767, 1978
21. Moss HB: More cases of anorgasmia after MAOI treatment (letter). *Am J Psychiatry* 140:266, 1983
22. Langs R: Psychoanalytic Psychotherapy, Vol. 1. New York: Jason Aronson, 1973, pp. 214–215
23. Mandell AJ: Psychoanalysis and psychopharmacology. In *Modern Psychoanalysis*, edited by Marmor J. New York: Basic Books, 1968
24. Marks IM: "Psycholopharmacology": the use of drugs combined with psychological treatment. In *Evaluation of Psychological Therapies*, edited by Spitzer RL, Klein DF. Baltimore: Johns Hopkins University Press, 1976
25. Mavissakalian M: Pharmacological treatment of anxiety disorders. *J Clin Psychiatry* 43:487–491

A Physician, a Nonmedical Psychotherapist, and a Patient: The Pharmacotherapy-Psychotherapy Triangle

John A. Chiles, Albert S. Carlin, and Bernard D. Beitman

The psychiatric research literature contains strong evidence to suggest the combination of psychotherapy and pharmacotherapy is useful in depression, schizophrenia, and anxiety states. The research literature also supports combined treatment in a variety of other disorders, eg, alcoholism, polydrug abuse, and anorexia nervosa. Comprehensive reviews of many of these indications are contained elsewhere in this book. While many psychiatrists provide their patients with both psychotherapy and pharmacotherapy, these modalities are sometimes delivered by different individuals. In this chapter we review the results of a survey addressing these triangular relationships and then outline issues relevant to their conduct.

QUESTIONNAIRE SURVEY

In an effort to determine the prevalence of psychologists and psychiatrists who see patients in combined psychotherapy and pharmacotherapy, we mailed questionnaires to members of the Washington State Psychiatric Association (387 members), to members of the Washington State Psychological Association, and to psychologists who are residents of Washington and members of the American Psychological Association (600 psychologists in all). Of the questionnaires mailed to psychiatrists, 217 (56 percent) were returned. Of the 600 questionnaires mailed to psychologists, 275 (46 percent) were returned. Of the psychologists returning the questionnaires, 193 could not be identified as licensed doctoral level clinical psychologists.

Sixty-three percent of the responding psychiatrists saw at least one pharmacotherapy patient during the month before receiving the questionnaire who was involved in psychotherapy with someone else. The median number of pharmacotherapy patients who were receiving psychotherapy from someone else was three while the mean was ten, suggesting that the majority of those psychiatrists treating patients in a triangular relationship see, at most, two or three per month while a few psychiatrists see a great many more, probably while working in an agency. Those psychiatrists treating patients in psychotherapy with someone else are younger, have been in practice fewer years, and are less likely to characterize themselves as psychoanalysts.

Among psychologists returning the questionnaire, approximately 79 percent provide psychotherapy for patients who are receiving psychoactive drugs. As can be seen from Table 2, psychologists who

Table 1.   Comparing Psychiatrists Who See Pharmacotherapy Patients in Triangles with Those Who Do Not

Mean age:	46.2 vs 51.0	p = 0.002
Mean years of practice:	12.3 vs 18.0	p = 0.001
Orientation — Psychoanalytic tended not to participate versus eclectic and psychodynamic who did:		p = 0.001

Table 2. Comparing Psychologists Who See Psychotherapy Patients in Triangles with Those Who Do Not

Mean age	43.4 vs 46.5	p = 0.08
Mean year of PhD	71.3 vs 68.2	p <0.05
Mean hours/week of psychotherapy	23.3 vs 8.8	p <0.001

see patients in combined treatment tend to be younger, have received their degrees more recently, and have relatively more extensive clinical practices. They are as likely to initiate referrals to pharmacotherapists as they are to receive referrals from pharmacotherapists.

These data indicate that treatment triangles are frequently formed. Nonphysician psychotherapists cannot prescribe drugs, and therefore need physicians for their medication-taking patients. They are increasingly aware of the efficacy of psychopharmacology treatments. On the other hand, a physician can deliver both modes of therapy, but may find that the limitations of time and knowledge prevent him/her from doing so. Medication management involves an awareness of internal medicine; the psychopharmacological literature can occupy much of one's professional reading time. Psychotherapy is increasingly specific, with increasingly more information available in interpersonal/family therapy, group therapy, various forms of cognitive/behavior, and the psychodynamic therapy. Many psychiatrists are now basing their practice on a knowledge of diagnosis, pharmacology, psychosomatic interplay, and a more thorough physical understanding of the patient [1-3]. They will assess and then manage the medication of patients doing psychotherapeutic work with other professionals. A physician can refer to nonmedical psychotherapists, or vice versa. The result is a three-way therapeutic interaction and contract. This "therapeutic triangle" if attended to, can provide the patient with a richer treatment program, infused with ideas from two different perspectives and academic backgrounds. This chapter reviews a number of aspects of the psychotherapy/pharmacotherapy triangle. We begin with the format: how to set one up, and what guidelines to follow.

INITIATION OF THE TRIANGLE

Success in a triangular relationship is enhanced by attention to detail. The patient must have not only an individual contract with each therapist, but also a contract for all three participants, spelling out such matters as the time and place the therapists and/or patient will meet to discuss the triangular arrangement, the fee for such a meeting, and its goals. Each therapist should maintain a set of written records for his/her individual work. A format for recording events in the three-way contract should also be worked out. Generally, we recommend that the therapist initiating the three-way action take responsibility for writing notes on the triangular contract throughout the course of treatment, and send a copy of these notes to the other therapist. A basic rule in establishing triangular arrangements is that the current therapist should never commit the other therapist to a course of treatment. A patient should never be told that he/she will be given medication or psychotherapy. A referral should always be something like, "this might be a good idea, let's see what my colleague thinks."

Ideally, the patient and both therapists meet to clarify the triangular arrangement. Although the therapists may be quite comfortable with one another, there is no substitute for face-to-face contact to establish the rules, especially in the patient's mind. Consider the situation in which the nonmedical therapist in initiating the triangular arrangement. He contacts the psychopharmacologist, gives a case description, and receives an initial impression about possible medications. The MD then meets and evaluates the patient and, if medication is appropriate, has the option of starting treatment and setting up a schedule for monitoring and follow-up. At this point, the initial three-way interview may be set up. The therapists should agree on the time, place, and fee for this meeting and the referring therapist should notify the patient.

DISCUSS THE REASONS FOR BOTH THERAPIES

Each therapist should attempt to let the patient know his/her role differences and similarities. This orientation reduces confusion, establishes a format for keeping objectives clear during treatment, and increases each therapist's ability to work toward compliance with the total plan. Usually, the referring therapist initiates the discussion by presenting the patient with a model of psychopathology and of treatment. The problem, or illness, or syndrome, should be discussed in ways which integrate biological and psychological mechanisms. These explanations should be tailored to the patient's explanatory model or personal theory of the disease [4]. The reviews of combined therapy in other chapters of this book may provide data for this discussion. The therapists may emphasize to the patient that the success of any therapy is dependent on a good initial evaluation and on continuous gathering of information. Introducing this idea early in the discussion may help in handling the crucial issue of confidentiality.

The issue of combining medication and psychotherapy may be approached in a general way. For example, "Medication can relieve many of the symptoms of anxiety and depression. You may notice increasing energy or clarity in your thinking. However, medications do not teach you new behaviors, and they do not change interpersonal situations. These areas may be approached by psychotherapy." This introduction makes sense to most patients, and may lead to a more explicit discussion of the treatment plan.

REVIEW INDIVIDUAL CONTRACTS

The review of individual contracts can be handled briefly. Each therapist should state the frequency of contact and estimate the duration of treatment in his/her modality. Pharmacotherapy often involves more intense initial evaluation, followed by infrequent checks as efficacy and adverse effects are well established. Psychotherapy often requires more frequent meetings over a longer period of time.

REVIEW TRIANGULAR CONTRACT

Confidentiality is a crucial issue for the treatment triangle. The therapists must be free to discuss any aspects of the case with one another; an envelope of confidentiality now encloses three, not two people. New ideas may occur to patient or therapist at any time, and patients may, for a variety of reasons, give information to one therapist but not to another. Patients may be offered an example or two here. For example:

A 62-year-old man began therapy with a clinical psychologist because of depression. His spouse had died six months earlier. Because he noted vegetative signs of depression, the psychologist obtained psychiatric consultation. The psychiatrist prescribed an antidepressant medication and both the therapists outlined the parameters of confidentiality. Later, the patient told the psychologist he was worried about his drinking. He had denied alcohol difficulties during his medical evaluation. The psychiatrist was told, and discussed drug-alcohol interactions with the patient. Alcohol management became part of the treatment for both therapists. The patient's reluctance to discuss alcohol with the physician was based on a past experience with another physician who had become "extremely angry" with him when he reported his drinking.

If need be, the patient can be assured that while all information is open to exchange, most of what the patient brings up will not be discussed in detail between the therapists. Each therapist needs to know the other's general impression of how the patient is doing and what changes in treatment plan have occurred. They are likely to discuss in greater detail problems of mutual concern like the alcoholism of the patient in the previous case. The therapists should also consider having regular contact with one another during the joint treatment. This communication can be done face-to-face, by phone, or by note, depending on the circumstances. The patient should know the schedule for this contract, and what additional fee, if any, is involved.

When a patient gives new information to one therapist, we encourage him/her to give it to the other, with the understanding that even if this does not happen, the therapists will talk about it in their next contact.

ISSUES OF JOINT CONCERN

Once the two therapies have been initiated, there will be many areas of overlap. One is universal—*compliance*; and another is fairly complex when it arises—the monitoring of *suicidal behavior*. Compliance is a troublesome issue in any health care delivery system. Securing a patient's active participation in a treatment program is an important task in any psychotherapeutic endeavor. Fortunately, the most direct way to do this is also the most efficacious [5]. Patients should be asked, in a friendly and helpful manner, whether or not they are following the guidelines of the treatment plan. Questions may be relatively simple: "Are you taking your medications as directed?" "How is your job hunting going?" "Are you and your spouse finding some time each day to practice new sexual techniques?" To do this effectively, the therapists must understand and accept the total treatment plan. Each therapist needs to adopt a "cheerleading," supportive stance toward the work of the other. In each session, each therapist may consider asking about progress, praising compliance, and encouraging continuation of the treatment program. If the patient is not following the treatment plan, then some inquiry is necessary. When hearing the patient's report of some outrageous act by the other therapist, each therapist should avoid the impulse to grimace, make a fist, or say "He did what? That's terrible!" What follows are two examples of these discussions; the psychotherapist reviewing pharmacotherapy, and the pharmacotherapist reviewing the psychotherapy.

PhD: How is your drug treatment going? Are you taking your medication as directed?

Pt: Well, some of the time.

PhD: I know it's hard to stick with a program day after day, but with this medication you must take it as directed. When you do not take it, what gets in the way?

Pt: I just forget. I am supposed to take it twice a day. Sometimes I miss one dose, sometimes I miss both doses.

PhD: That does happen, but fortunately, there are ways to help you remember. Any other reasons why you sometimes miss a dose?

Pt: Well, to tell the truth, this stuff makes my mouth dry and I don't like that.

PhD: That may be a side effect of the medication, and it is important to talk to Dr. Jones about both the dry mouth and ways of remembering to take the medicine. What you need to do is make a special effort to take the pills as directed, and bring up both these points in your next meeting with Dr. Jones. I will be sure to mention to him that you have these two concerns.

And:

MD: How is your psychotherapy going?

Pt: So-so.

MD: Are you having some difficulties with it?

Pt: It's Dr. Smith. She seems kind of cold. Not like you. You seem to understand me better.

MD: Psychotherapy can stir up strong emotions. Please consider discussing your feelings over with Dr. Smith. It may be hard, but talking about negative feelings often leads to good results in the kind of therapeutic work you are doing. I'll be checking with her in two weeks. My hunch is you'll be glad you talked over these emotions with her.

Please notice, especially in the second example, that the colleague is supported, splitting is avoided, and an issue that may involve transference problems is referred, in a positive way, to the appropriate therapist.

The *suicidal* patient is often most difficult. There is no current pharmacological treatment for suicidal behavior, although several interesting avenues are currently under investigation [6]. However, suicidal behavior is found in patients with a variety of psychiatric illnesses and these illnesses are often treated by pharmacologic means. The disorder most frequently associated with suicidal behavior is depression; this diagnosis is made 28 percent of the time among male suicide attempters, and 40 percent of the time among female suicide attempters [7].

Suicidal behavior has also been reported in increased frequency with anxiety disorders, especially when they are associated with panic attacks [8]. Both anxiety and depression are likely to respond to pharmacological intervention. This fact is troublesome since antianxiety agents and antidepressant agents are frequently used in deliberate overdose; however, the frequency of suicide in psychiatric patients [9] is low enough that it should not interfere with effective treatment. If a patient has suicidal ideation, and/or has a past history of suicide attempts, these issues should be addressed in the triangular meeting. The therapists should emphasize that no medication works unless it is taken as directed. Many suicide attempters are impulsive, and this characteristic should be addressed as an important issue for psychotherapy. The patient and both therapists should agree upon a contract for a reasonable period of time, perhaps six weeks in the case of antidepressants, during which the medication is to be taken as directed and not to be used in any self-destructive way. Many patients will cooperate with a time-limited contract which looks for potential benefits from medication. They will respond less well to medication prescribed for an indefinite period of time and for vague reasons. As noted before, nonmedical therapists can help by asking about compliance. Additionally, both therapists should monitor suicidal ideation and behavior and be alert to the hints the patient is sequestering medication. Careful notes about these discussions are essential. Potentially suicidal patients should be given frequent prescriptions containing nonlethal amounts of medication. Whether prescriptions for these small amounts are handled by the psychotherapist in the regular weekly meeting or by increased frequency of meeting with the pharmacotherapist is a question to be negotiated.

Patients often suffer from pharmacologically treatable psychiatric illness and also have troublesome personality traits, as discussed by Ward in Chapter 3. These personality traits must be taken into account in relationship development and compliance enhancement. The therapists should consider discussing these traits, and develop a "party line" approach so that the patient will find some consistency in each therapist's style. A dependent patient may respond best to a warm and somewhat global explanation about recommendations, while an obsessive patient might need extensive detail, and might view warmth suspiciously. One patient may be able to collaborate fully and do well with a flexible approach. Another may respond best to a high degree of authority. Therapists consulting about their approaches to a patient often get to know each other a little better and do some mutual teaching. Usually, differences of opinion about approaches to a patient can either be resolved or understood and tolerated.

EMERGENCIES

In the initial meeting, the possibility of emergencies should be raised. Each therapist should develop a way of handling emergencies in their individual work, and these procedures should be explained to the patient. At times, the therapist who should handle a specific emergency is obvious. For example, interpersonal disruptions are often best handled in the context of the ongoing psychotherapy, while extrapyramidal reactions to the antipsychotic medication are clearly in the province of the psychopharmacotherapist. Other situations are less clear. For example, a sudden feeling of dysphoria and confusion could have one of many causes. Patients are not required to sort out responsibilities in the case of emergencies and should be permitted to contact either therapist. If hospitalization is an issue, the psychiatrist is usually more likely to handle the decision.

OTHER ISSUES

A host of other issues may enter the triangular arrangement and may need to be stated explicitly in the contract. If supervision is involved, the patient may be informed, told why, and understand his/her responsibility in the matter; ie, will he/she be charged for the time? Is either therapist expecting the other to provide coverage for vacation? A pharmacotherapist who has been meeting with a patient for 15 minutes a month may be startled when suddenly being told by a patient that the psychotherapist is out of town for two weeks and he/she would like an hour appointment to "talk things over." Vacation coverage can be a helpful addition to a triangular relationship, giving the patient a familiar person as back-up, but the arrangement must be spelled out beforehand.

Couples in therapy present a special problem to triangular arrangements. Some times, as couples engage in psychotherapy, one of the pair develops psychiatric symptoms, and receives a referral for pharmacotherapy. While medication may be useful, it also may invalidate, in the nonmedicated spouse's mind, the usefulness of the couple's work. "Now, clearly, I can see that it's not me, it's him (or her). He is sick, and needs medication." When a couple is in ongoing therapy, the psychopharmacotherapist should consider seeing both patients initially. Medication should be discussed in the context of the couple's work. The couple should also be included in the triangular interview, and the therapists' ideas about the efficacy of psychotherapy and pharmacotherapy spelled out. The danger of seeing one member of a couple initially involves confidentiality. For example:

A couple had been in psychotherapy with a counselor for approximately four months. During this time, the wife had become increasingly withdrawn. Her husband reported that she seemed distracted and depressed, and wasn't "her old self." She was referred to a pharmacotherapist for evaluation of depression. She started this session by telling the pharmacotherapist that she was feeling fine, and that she was having an affair. This affair was unknown to her husband, and she did not want him told. The pharmacotherapist now knew more than he wanted to about the couple's relationship, especially without any clear and agreed upon means of transmitting this information to the other therapist.

Table 3. Sources of Referral to Psychologists of Patients Seen Jointly in Psychotherapy and Pharmacotherapy

	Percentage
Same agency	21
Same building	16
Share office	11
Same network	9
Friends	26
Spouse	0
Previous referrals	72

Triangular contracts are also influenced by timing, ie, when in the course of the patient's overall treatment they are set up. One variable is the therapists' familiarity with each other. As therapists become more comfortable and knowledgeable about one another, triangular arrangements seem to be initiated earlier in treatment. The referring therapist develops a quicker sense that his/her colleague will be useful, and initiates the process. The further along in time a patient is in one mode of therapy, the potentially more complex is the addition of a second therapist, especially when the first therapist feels stuck or frustrated. Referral for consultation may offer an effective way out of troubled waters, but also may seem to be a withdrawal or rejection. Sometimes the request for a consultation does mean more than a request for a treatment triangle. Instead it may be a latent request to transfer an undesirable patient.

Table 4. Referral Resources for Pharmacotherapy for Psychologists Who See Patients Seen Jointly

	Percentage
Same agency	23
Same building	10
Same office	12
Same network	7
Friends	21
Spouse	1
Previous referrals	66

Sometimes the referring therapist may be asking for psychotherapy supervision, not medications.

The triangular relationship requires openness, trust, the ability to diplomatically contact a colleague on a puzzling treatment decision, and to tolerate being questioned about one's own treatment decision. Given the complexities of this triangular relationship, it is not surprising that the most common referral sources are friends and those with whom previous referral relationships have been successful (Tables 3 and 4). A number of respondents to our survey questionnaires indicated that when they have experienced difficulties with a referral source or resource they simply faded their professional relationship with that individual. Therapists (psycho- or pharmaco-) who are indirect, unprofessional, or selfish will find themselves involved in fewer and fewer therapeutic triangles.

Our findings indicate that collaborative arrangements between psychotherapists and pharmacotherapists are common and for the most part, work well. These arrangements should be viewed as unique opportunities to enhance compliance to therapeutic plans rather than situations in which patients are likely to sabotage both treatments.

ACKNOWLEDGMENTS

This work was supported in part by a Biomedical Research Support Grant #61-2837, University of Washington. Computational assistance was provided by CLINFO computer systems funded under General Clerical Research Center Grant #RR-37.

REFERENCES

1. Winslow W: The changing role of psychiatrists in community mental health centers. *Am J Psychiatry* 136:24–27, 1979
2. Pardes H: Future needs for psychiatrists and other mental health personnel. *Arch Gen Psychiatry* 36:1401–1408, 1979
3. McIntyre JS, Romano J: Is there a stethoscope in the house (and is it used)? *Arch Gen Psychiatry* 34:1147–1151, 1977
4. Katon W: Doctor-patient negotiation and other social science strategies in patient care. In *The Relevance of Social Science for Medicine*, edited by Eisenberg L, Kleinman A. Dordrecht, Holland: D. Reidel Publishing Co, 1981, pp. 253–279

5. Haynes RB, Taylor DW, Sackett DL (eds): *Compliance in Health Care.* Baltimore: Johns Hopkins University Press, 1979
6. Montgomery SA, Montgomery D: Pharmacological prevention of suicidal behavior. *J Affective Disord* 4:291-298, 1982
7. Kreitman N: *Parasuicide.* London: Wiley, 1977
8. Coryell W, Noyes R, Clancy J: Excesses mortality in panic disorder. *Arch Gen Psychiatry* 39:701-703, 1982
9. Pokorny AD: Prediction of suicide in psychiatric patients. *Arch Gen Psychiatry* 40:249-257, 1983

PART III
Specific Diagnostic Categories

CHAPTER 6

Research Considerations in Evaluating Combined Treatments

Gerald L. Klerman

INTRODUCTION

The chapters in this section discuss the research evidence and clinical experience with combined treatments for four clinical conditions: depression, schizophrenia, agoraphobia and panic disorder, and anorexia nervosa. The selection of these conditions does not exhaust the range of possibilities. A comprehensive survey would include reports on the possible value of combined treatment for many other conditions; bipolar affective disorder, obsessive-compulsive states, obesity, bulimia, and borderline personality disorder, to list a few. However, these four conditions were selected because they are of public health importance and societal concern, as well as clinically significant.

These conditions represent areas of considerable research activity. The drugs and psychotherapies employed in combined treatment include a variety of modalities, including tricyclic antidepressants and neuroleptics among the drug treatments, and cognitive, interpersonal, family, and behavioral treatments among the psychotherapies. A large number of controlled clinical trials have been conducted to assess the efficacy of combined treatment and the design, execution and data analysis of the research reported in the chapters are representative of the "state of the art" in current research on clinical therapeutics.

Diagnosis and the Medical Model

One feature of the chapters in this section merits special attention—the use of diagnostic category as the basis for selection of patients for the clinical treatment research programs. Diagnosis has always been the criteria for selection of patients for drug studies. One of the major characteristics of the "new wave" of psychotherapy research is the growing acceptance of the concept of multiple mental disorders and increasing attention to the importance of diagnosis and classification. These characteristics are evident in the development of psychotherapies for specific disorders, for example, cognitive-behavioral and interpersonal psychotherapies for depression, desensitization and exposure-in-vivo for agoraphobia, and family therapy directed at reducing expressed-emotions (EE) in families of discharged schizophrenics. Furthermore, the research projects now employ structured interviews for collection information about history and symptoms and research criteria for making diagnoses.

These trends represent a departure from previous periods when classification and diagnosis were rejected and patients were selected for psychotherapy, particularly psychodynamic psychotherapy, not on the basis of symptoms and diagnosis, but on the basis of personality characteristics, such as ego strength, defensive structure, or conflict area.

The use of diagnosis in the design and conduct of research on psychotherapy either alone or in combination with drugs, places psychotherapy in the health care system. In other contexts, one might say "in the medical model," but in addition to concern for diagnosis and classification, the medical model in mental health often includes three other elements: (1) professional domination by physicians, including psychiatrists, (2) biological explanations of causation, and (3) exclusive reliance on somatic forms of treatment. Since all these components are controversial for purposes of reducing controversy and enhancing understanding and communication, I focus on the relationship of psychotherapy to the health care system [1].

Viewing psychotherapy as a health procedure legitimizes reimbursement by health insurance and other third-party providers independent of whether the psychotherapy is delivered by a medical person or whether biological factors are considered etiologic for the disorder. For example, biofeedback, relaxation, exercise, and control of diet are all behavioral and psychotherapeutic interventions of value for patients with hypertension, a biological disorder with adverse health consequences.

Critics have pointed out that there are possible adverse consequences for the sick role and for seeing psychotherapy as a health procedure. It is argued that whatever short-term benefits may come, are at the expense of enhancing the patient's dependency and promoting the sick role behavior. From a psychodynamic point of view, this is often regarded as a form of manipulating the transference, particularly to enhance the physician being seen as a transference object who is authoritarian, paternalistic, enhancing dependency, and promoting regressive if not infantile reliance on the physician and the health care system. In behavioral terms, the concern is that there will be reinforcement of the sick role behavior, particularly those aspects of the sick role which excuse the individual from responsibility and may reinforce avoidant behavior. Biological psychiatrists often argue that it is inappropriate to regard psychotherapy as a health procedure not only because of the alleged lack of efficacy, but more importantly because of their view that the only legitimate interventions are those of a biological nature, via medications, electroconvulsive therapy, or other somatic treatments.

These considerations, however, only increase the need for research to assess the efficacy and safety of these health-related interventions. Future research may not support the value of developing disorder-specific treatments. Research may demonstrate that patient personality or therapist characterization are more powerful predictors of response to psychotherapy than symptom-pattern or diagnosis. However, without appropriate research, these conflicting claims and assertions perpetuate ideological tension and impair the credibility of psychotherapy with patients and policy-makers.

RESEARCH DESIGNS FOR EVALUATING TREATMENTS ALONE AND IN COMBINATION

Ideally, before combined treatments are employed, four types of evidence should be available: (1) evidence for the efficacy of each treatment modality, (2) understanding of the mechanism of actions of the two treatments, (3) verified concepts of the nature of the disorder that bridge the two treatments and provide a reasonable basis for the combination, and (4) evidence for the efficacy of the combination. This ideal is seldom realized in medicine in general, let alone in psychiatry. Most psychiatric treatments, including psychotherapy and pharmacotherapy, are derived inductively from serendipity and experience rather than "rationally" from deductions from an established body of knowledge.

Nevertheless, the value of many treatments are accepted even if the etiology or pathophysiology of the disorder is uncertain or the mechanism of action of the treatment is not established. For scientific, clinical practice, evidence for (1) and (4) are necessary, and (2) and (3), while desirable, are not always present [2].

The Importance of the Randomized Controlled Trial

It is now generally agreed that the most powerful evidence for the efficacy of any health intervention, including treatments of any sort—pharmacologic, surgical, radiation, or psychological, comes from the randomized controlled clinical trial. This design has been most widely employed for evaluating drugs but it is increasingly being used with other forms of treatment, including psychotherapies.

Although the theoretical basis for the randomized trial goes back to writings on scientific investigation in the 17th century, the first applications in medical therapeutics did not appear until the 20th century with the development of placebo-control trials. However, the impetus for increasing application of randomized controlled trials came from public concern and legislative mandate.

In the US, the crucial event occurred in 1962, when the Kefauver-Harris Amendments to the Food and Drug Act were enacted. For the first time, evidence for efficacy was required before the approval of a new drug. Today, we take the criteria of safety and efficacy for granted in the health field. However, these criteria were mandated only after a hard-fought Congressional battle. Before 1962, evidence for efficacy was not required for the marketing of new pharmaceutic

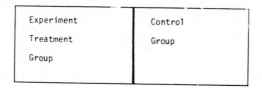

Figure 1.   Two-group design.

products. Safety was mandated in 1938 legislation, but until that time, only evidence of purity, provided for in the 1908 legislation, was required.

Interestingly, safety and efficacy criteria are not included in other Federal statutes for any other health programs. For example, they are not required for Medicare or Medicaid reimbursement. The statute stipulates that reimbursement procedures be "necessary and reasonable." There is currently a vigorous debate in Washington over proposals that would extend the criteria of efficacy to psychiatric treatment, such as psychotherapy [3].

Establishing the Efficacy of a Single Treatment

To evaluate a single treatment, such as a new drug or form of psychotherapy, the minimum design is a two-group design, as shown in Figure 1, in which the new treatment is compared with some appropriate control group. In the case of pharmacotherapy, the usual control group is a placebo. In the case of the psychotherapies, there remains controversy as to what is the equivalent of the placebo as the control group.

A more optimal design for evaluating a new treatment is a three-group design in which the new treatment is compared against some standard treatment, as well as a control (Figure 2). Thus, in a study of a new antidepressant, it is desirable to compare the new drug with a standard drug, such as imipramine or amitriptyline, and with a placebo. In the case of psychotherapy, where relatively few standard treatments exist, it is often considered useful to compare two forms of psychotherapy against a controlled group. For example, the NIMH Collaborative Study on the Psychotherapy of Depression is comparing cognitive therapy and interpersonal therapy with psychological management with placebo and imipramine, thereby expanding the three-group design to four-group design.

Experimental Treatment Group	Standard Treatment Group	Control Group

Figure 2.   Three-group design.

Evidence For Efficacy of Somatic Treatments

As stated earlier, the ideal situation for assessing the theoretical and therapeutic aspects of combined drug and psychotherapy would be to possess the empirical evidence on the efficacy of each of these therapies. The assumption in combining treatments is that independent studies will have shown efficacy for the drug and for the psychotherapy over a control group.

The available evidence on drug treatments is extensive and generally confirms their efficacy and safety [4]. There is little doubt that clinical practices for treating affective disorders were revolutionized in the late 1950s by the introduction of the antidepressant drugs—tricyclics and monoamine oxidase inhibitors (MAOIs)—and lithium. Their effectiveness in clinical practice has been documented in a number of well-controlled clinical trials. For symptom relief and resolution of acute depressive episodes, the antidepressants have demonstrated efficacy. In addition, there is now substantial evidence for the value of two classes of drugs for maintenance therapy to prevent relapse and recurrence: lithium for bipolar and unipolar recurrent depressions and tricyclics for unipolar recurrent depression only.

Evidence for Efficacy of Psychotherapies

I use the term "psychotherapy" in a very broad sense to include psychoanalysis, psychotherapy, counseling, forms of behavior modification, reassurance, and other regimens. There is no single psychotherapy, just as there is no one drug.

For decades, scientists and clinicians have questioned the usefulness of psychotherapy [5,6], but recent reports provide increasingly convincing evidence for the therapeutic effects of psychotherapy in general. For affective disorders in particular, the evidence for the efficacy of psychotherapy is growing but is not yet as conclusive as that for drug therapy. Because the prevalence rates for depression are higher than for other types of affective disorders, most of the available research assessing the efficacy of psychotherapy has been conducted using depressed outpatients. Advances in nosology, better specification of treatments, improved scientific designs, and higher standards for conducting clinical trials have resulted in a sufficient number of studies so that assessment of the evidence is now possible [7].

Weissman [8] reviewed the evidence for the efficacy of psychotherapy alone and in comparison with and combination with pharmacotherapy for the treatment of depression. She documented the dramatic increase in the quantity and quality of the evidence during the 1970s and identified 17 clinical trials that tested the efficacy of five types of psychotherapies—behavioral, cognitive, group, interpersonal, and marital—in depressed outpatients.

To examine the data from the perspective of the psychotherapies as a group, Weissman looked at data from the nine studies that specifically tested the efficacy of psychotherapy in comparison with a low-contact or no-active-treatment control group. All nine studies supported the efficacy of psychotherapy alone as compared with a control group [8]. Five treatment approaches were represented. Studies using cognitive therapy were described by Rush and Beck [9] and by Rush et al [10], behavior therapy was tested by Rehm [11], interpersonal psychotherapy was tested by Klerman et al [12] and Weissman et al [8], and studies testing group and marital therapy were reported by Covi et al [13] and Friedman [14].

Establishing the Efficacy of Combined Treatments

When one wishes to evaluate a combined treatment, such as the combination of two drugs (a tricyclic plus benzodiazepine) or the combination of a drug plus psychotherapy (amitriptyline plus interpersonal therapy), the minimum design is the four-group design. In the four-group design, each treatment is evaluated against each other, against a control group, and against the combination.

However, when evaluating the combination of drugs and psychotherapy, a number of additional problems arise as a consequence of the placebo effect. The usual setting for psychotherapy does not involve use of a placebo. Some observers have argued that even taking an inert substance alters the sociopsychological context of the psychotherapy, especially by generating changes in expectations, both of the therapist and of the patient. Therefore, the more

		DRUG TREATMENT	
		Experimental Treatment	Control Treatment
PSYCHOTHERAPY	Experimental Treatment	Combined Treatment Group	Psychotherapy Treatment Group
	Control Treatment	Drug Treatment Group	Control Group

Figure 3.   Four-group design for evaluating combined treatment.

powerful design would be a six-group design. This design was used in a trial of drugs and psychotherapy in maintenance treatment of acute depressions reported by Klerman et al [12].

The six group design tests whether or not there was a placebo variable or increment over and above the nonspecific conditions of numerous rating scales and of the illness itself. There seems to be an assumption implicit in much of the placebo literature that the placebo effect is positive in all conditions and in all circumstances. Most of the literature on placebo groups deals with the specific expectations around pill taking—its so-called magical and dependency expectation—and a whole host of other nonspecific factors, such as being given the "sick role" and the special attention of being in a research project. In the Boston-New Haven study, we did not find any placebo effect over and above the "no-pill" condition in a long-term (eight-month) treatment study of depressive patients. We did find a drug versus "no-pill" and drug versus placebo difference, but we could not detect any placebo effect over and above the "no-pill" condition in that study. No negative interactions between drugs and psychotherapy were observed [15].

Hollon [16] proposes that a more optimal design for studying the interaction of drugs and psychotherapy would be a nine-cell design to control for the nonspecific or placebo aspects of psychotherapy. No one has yet attempted a nine-cell design, and to our knowledge there is only one six-cell design. A number of four-cell design projects have been reported, and this gives some data base for the assessment of the efficacy of combined treatment.

		PSYCHOTHERAPY	
		Present	Absent
DRUG TREATMENT	Drug	Psychotherapy Plus Drug Group	Drug Group
	Placebo	Psychotherapy Plus Placebo Group	Placebo Group
	No Pill	Psychotherapy Group	No Pill No Psychotherapy

Figure 4. Six-group design for evaluating placebo-effect in combined treatment.

POSSIBLE OUTCOMES OF COMBINED TREATMENT

Having defined some of the possible designs, let us now analyze the possible outcomes, using as a basis for discussion, the four-group design as shown in Figure 3. The graphs assume that minimal methodologic criteria are met: predetermined criteria for selection, randomization or some other form of systematic assignment to the experimental and control groups, predetermined quantitative measures of outcome, and some degree of blindness on the part of the observers as to which treatment the subjects or patients are receiving.

The assumption in almost all drug studies is that the drug-treated group will show a greater degree of improvement over the control group (usually a placebo group). In research of behavioral or psychotherapy interventions, this design has been a source of controversy regarding both its appropriations and difficulty in execution. Numerous debates have arisen over the appropriate outcome measures, the nature of the placebo, or the appropriate control group in psychotherapy research.

In Figures 5 through 8, the height of the bars representing treatment outcome is equal for both the psychotherapy and the drug groups. This reflects an attempt to be fair regarding the two forms of

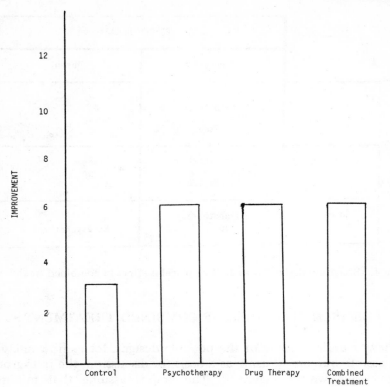

Figure 5. Combined treatment outcome: no therapeutic effect.

treatment. For example, in studies of depression, Rush and Beck [9] have published evidence from a two-cell design that cognitive therapy is equal to efficacy to treatment with a tricyclic. Their finding has challenged the conventional wisdom within the depression field, which has assumed that drugs would have more impact than any behavioral or psychotherapeutic intervention.

Assuming the minimal four-cell design, what are the possible outcomes? I have catalogued the possible outcomes of the relationship of the combined cell to the two individual treatments. In Figures 5 through 8, the left bar refers to the control group, the middle bars refer to the two active therapies of pharmacotherapy, and the bar on the right refers to the combined treatment.

At least three types of interaction outcomes are discussed in the literature:

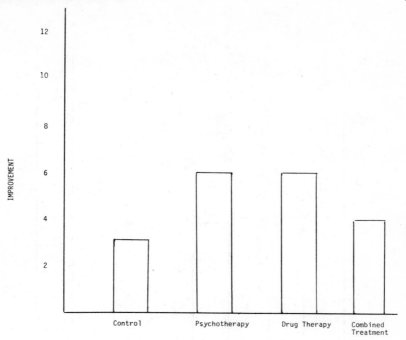

Figure 6. Combined treatment outcome: negative therapeutic effect.

1. *No Therapeutic Effect* (Figure 5): Combined treatment provides the same improvement as the individual treatments.

2. *Negative Effect* (Figure 6): Combined treatment shows less improvement than the effect of either treatment alone.

3. *Additive Effect* (Figure 7): Combined treatment enhances the effect of either treatment alone.

No therapeutic effect of combination is reported in Figure 5, in which the effect of combined treatment offers no greater benefit than single treatments, both of which are better than control. Ideally and optimistically, we hope for some additive effects (Figure 7) in which the sum is greater than its parts—that the combined treatment will produce a magnitude of effect greater than the two individual treatments.

I have reviewed the literature to find examples of each type of outcome. The most common reports are of some degree of

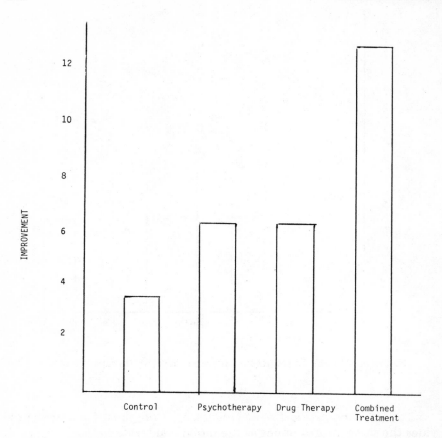

Figure 7. Combined treatment outcome: additive effect.

additive effect, and that the combined treatments offer better results than either treatment alone.

The ideal additive effects would be synergistic, such that the effect of combined treatment is greater than the sum of the two component treatments. This has occurred in the Boston-New Haven Project on the treatment of acute outpatient depressive patients. In this study, the outcome measure utilized was the Hamilton Depressive Scale.

Finally, there is the complex pattern of what I shall call "facilitation" intervention. As shown in Figure 8, one of the

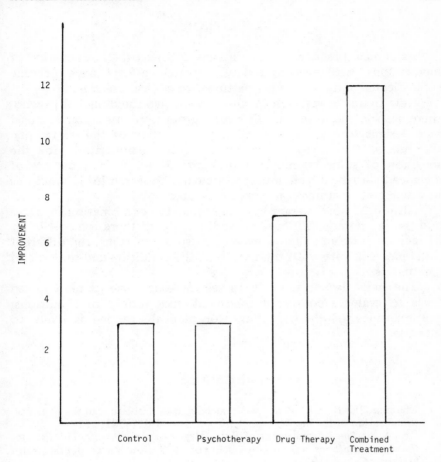

Figure 8. Combined treatment outcomes: complex facilitative effect.

treatments is ineffective alone, but the combination is most effective. This is the outcome reported for most studies with schizophrenia; the psychotherapy alone is ineffective but when combined with pharmacotherapy, some additive effect occurs. This complex facilitative effect is implicit in clinical practice with bipolar patients, psychotic depressed patients, and melancholic (or endogenous) depressed patients. Psychotherapy alone is ineffective. Patients with this diagnosis require medication, and the combined treatment offers advantage.

CONCLUSIONS

As clinical practice has increasingly involved the combination of medications with psychotherapy, research efforts have become sophisticated and increasingly pertinent to clinical practice.

New trends in research in this area involve the design of psychotherapies specific to various diagnostic groups, the use of randomized trial designs to evaluate the efficacy and safety of the treatments, the use of structured interviews and diagnostic criteria for the selection of subjects, multiple outcome measures, and the use of advanced statistical techniques, particularly to search for interactions in which two treatments are being evaluated.

Although most therapists assume that the combination of drugs and psychotherapy will have an additive effect, there is a possibility of lack of interactions and even negative interactions; the different outcomes will vary with the nature of the condition and the type of treatments.

The next decade is likely to see increasing use of randomized trials to evaluate combined treatment in a variety of conditions; the relevance of these findings for clinical practice is likely to increase.

REFERENCES

1. Klerman GL: Better but not well: social and ethical issues in the deinstitutionalization of the mentally ill. *Schizophr Bull* 3:617-631, 1977
2. Group for The Advancement of Psychiatry: *Pharmacotherapy and Psychotherapy: Paradoxes and Progress.* 9:Report #93. New York: Mental Health Materials Center, 1975
3. Klerman GL: The efficacy of psychotherapy as the basis for public policy. *Am Psychol* 38:929-934, 1983
4. Klein DF, Gittleman-Klein R: *Progress in Psychiatric Drug Treatment.* New York: Brunner/Mazel, 1976
5. Garfield SL, Bergin AE (eds): *Handbook of Psychiatry and Behavior Change,* 2nd ed. New York: John Wiley and Sons, 1978
6. Glass GV, Smith ML, Miller TI: *The Benefits of Psychotherapy.* Baltimore: Johns Hopkins University Press, 1980
7. Rush J, ed: *Short-Term Psychotherapies for Depression.* New York: The Guilford Press, 1982
8. Weissman MM: The psychological treatment of depression: research evidence for the efficacy of psychotherapy alone, in comparison and in combination with pharmacotherapy. *Arch Gen Psychiatry.* 36:1261-1269, 1979
9. Rush AJ, Beck AT: Behavior therapy in adults eith affective disorders. In: *Behavior Therapy in the Psychiatric Setting,* edited by Herson M, Bellack AS. Baltimore: Williams and Wilkins, 1980

10. Rush AJ, Beck AT, Kovacs M, et al: Comparative efficacy of cognitive therapy and pharmacotherapy in the treatment of depressed outpatients. *Cog Ther Res* 1:17–37, 1977
11. Rehm LP: Studies in self-control treatment of depression. Presented to the American Psychological Association, Washington, DC, September, 1976
12. Klerman, GL, DiMascio A, Weissman MM, et al: Treatment of depression by drugs and psychotherapy. *Am J Psychiatry* 131:186–191, 1974
13. Covi L, Lipman R, Derogatis L, et al: Drugs and group psychotherapy in neurotic depression. *Am J Psychiatry* 131:191–198, 1974
14. Friedman AS: Interaction of drug therapy with marital therapy in depressed patients. *Arch Gen Psychiatry* 32:619–637, 1975
15. Rounsaville BJ, Klerman GL, Weissman MM: Do psychotherapy and pharmacotherapy for depression conflict? *Arch Gen Psychiatry* 38:24–29, 1981
16. Hollon SD: Presentation at the 14th Annual Meeting of the Society for Psychotherapy Research, 1983

CHAPTER 7

Cognitive Therapy in Combination with Antidepressant Medication

A. John Rush

INTRODUCTION

This chapter summarizes the available research data on the indications for the combination of cognitive psychotherapy [1] and antidepressant pharmacotherapy. For the most part, these data are incomplete and provide only slight help to the clinician in making this important decision. After the summary of research data, clinically derived guidelines and case examples illustrate how I approach this question as a practitioner. In general, my approach has been to apply the scientific-empirical method to treatment planning for depressed patients. A carefully rendered descriptive psychiatric diagnosis is essential. Organic, medical, neurologic, and iatrogenic causes for depression are identified and treated. The affective disorder is subtyped (eg, bipolar, unipolar, endogenous or nonendogenous, etc). Then, a single intervention is typically applied—cognitive therapy or pharmacotherapy. Response and side effects are monitored. Maximal effort is placed on single treatment to maximize therapeutic effect. Should symptomatic remission ensue, then medication is maintained for six months and gradually discontinued. If medication-responsive patients have psychosocial, interpersonal, or psychological problems that persist after maximal medication benefit has been obtained, then psychotherapy directed at these drug nonresponsive problems is conducted. If the patient has only a partial response to medication, either the dose must be adjusted, the medication must be changed, or psychotherapy aimed at further symptom reduction is instituted. This particular choice can be difficult. However, the persistent presence of some endogenous symptom features (eg, anhedonia or unreactive mood, or insomnia) argue for modification of the medication regimen, whereas if those symptoms that persist are largely cognitive (eg, a negative view of self or world, or social avoidance) then the addition of cognitive therapy might be the preferred avenue.

For the patient with a nonendogenous, nonpsychotic unipolar depression, cognitive therapy may be the first treatment recommended. Again, symptom reduction, and, in fact, complete symptom remission, is the goal. If the patient responds fully, no medication is needed. A partial response leads me to review the differential diagnosis, and in many cases to then add antidepressant medication— again with the goal of complete symptomatic remission. In a few cases, I think both treatments are needed to obtain complete symptom remission as illustrated later.

DIAGNOSIS OF DEPRESSION

Perhaps the most crucial purpose of diagnosis is to improve the match of available treatments with the problems presented by each patient. A second purpose is prognostication—to help patients, relatives, and society at large to anticipate the most likely outcome of a particular medical problem. When diagnoses are based on signs and symptoms alone, one must take into account the fact that sex, age, and the patient's personality, as well as a host of other variables, may affect the presentation of a particular syndrome. When one turns to diagnosis based on course of illness, naturalistic studies of depressed patients are few and far between, and most are confounded with the

Table 1. Major Depressive Episode

A. Dysphoria or loss of interest/pleasure in all or almost all usual activities.

B. At least four present for two weeks:

1. Appetite/weight loss or gain
2. Sleep disturbance
3. Psychomotor changes
4. Loss of interest/pleasure or libido
5. Loss of energy, fatigue
6. Self-criticism (guilt or self-blame)
7. Decreased concentration, speed of thought, decision making
8. Recurrent thought of death, suicide or attempt

C. Picture not dominated by:

1. Mood-incongruent hallucinations/delusions, or
2. Bizarre behavior

D. Not superimposed on schizophrenia, schizophreniform or paranoid disorder

E. Not due to organic mental disorder of bereavement

currently available therapeutic interventions that may range from psychoanalysis or short-term psychotherapies to antidepressant medications or electroconvulsive therapy. While diagnosis based on treatment response may be of particular value for researchers, it does not allow the physician to select treatment for an individual patient.

In light of these problems, DSM-III [2] diagnoses are simply based on the apparent phenomenology (the specific signs and symptoms) without attempting to imply a specific etiology. Thus, the syndromes of major depression, dysthymia, mania, and hypomania have multiple etiologies.

DSM-III details the criteria employed for the diagnosis of nine different forms of affective disorders. The reader is referred to this volume for details [2]. Table 1 presents the criteria for major depression.

Figure 1 shows a flow chart or decision tree that can be employed clinically in the differential diagnosis of dysphoric patients. Dysphoria may be described by the patient as sadness, anxiety, irritability, or a combination of these affects. Most dysphorias in everyday life are tied to affective responses to daily life events. Such normal dysphorias are typically brief and lead neither to functional impairment nor to help-seeking from psychiatric or other medical professionals.

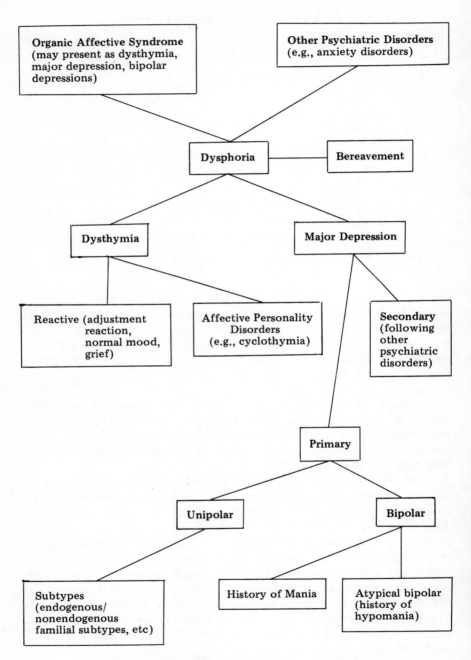

Figure 1.   The differential diagnosis of dysphoria.

On the other hand, a variety of medical disorders are also associated with dysphoria. Organic affective disorders can present as dysphoria, dysthymia, or major depression. In addition, grief or bereavement is typified by dysphoria, but grief is by definition a time-limited state that occurs in relation to the loss of a particularly important other person. If the symptomatology of a grieving patient persists more than six months after a loss, and meets the criteria for major depression, then major depression is the diagnosis.

While adjustment reactions may be accompanied by dysphoria, they do not meet the criteria for major depression or dysthymia. Once organic affective disorders, grief or bereavement, adjustment reactions, and medical illnesses associated with dysphoria are eliminated, one is left with the psychiatric affective disorders. Therefore, one may subdivide major depressions into the primary and secondary groups. Primary depression is diagnosed when no other major psychiatric syndrome except mania or depression precedes the onset of major depression. Secondary depressions are major depressions that are preceded by other major psychiatric syndromes such as alcoholism, schizophrenia, drug dependency, etc. Whether primary and secondary depression differ in their responsiveness to psychotherapy, chemotherapy, or the combination is unknown.

The endogenous/nonendogenous dichotomy is a classification initially based on etiology. Nonendogenous depressions were assumed to be responses to life problems, whereas endogenous depressions arose "from the inside." Recent data, however, indicate that most patients with endogenous depressions are likely to attribute cause to life events. Thus, the presence or absence of life stresses is no longer the critical differentiation of endogenous from nonendogenous depressions. Truly, "endogenous" depressions— meaning those depressions that occur without pre-existing life stresses—are relatively rare. Van Praag found that only 16 percent of 92 patients with endogenous depressions by clinical descriptive criteria failed to report either psychosocial or somatic stressors [3,4]. Subsequent studies have found no correlation between the nature of the stressor and the nature of the depressive syndrome [5]. Thus, stressors are not sufficient to cause depression, and a particular stressor does not provoke a particular depressive reaction [6].

Presently, the term endogenous refers to a symptom constellation detailed in the Research Diagnostic Criteria (RDC) [7]. DSM-III uses the term "melancholic" to refer to a similar group of patients that is more narrowly defined. Table 2 specifies the endogenous symptom criteria found in the RDC [7], and Table 3 lists melancholic symptom features as noted in DSM-III [2].

Table 2. Diagnostic Criteria for Endogenous Depression

One symptom from group A and a total of six symptoms from group A and B:

A.
1. Distinct quality to depressed mood
2. Lack of reactivity to environmental changes
3. Mood is regularly worse in the morning
4. Pervasive loss of interest or pleasure

B.
1. Feelings of self-reproach or excessive or inappropriate guilt
2. Early morning awakening or middle insomnia
3. Psychomotor retardation or agitation
4. Poor appetite
5. Weight loss
6. Loss of interest or pleasure in usual activities or decreased sexual drive

DSM-III criteria for depression with melancholic symptom features are similar, though more restrictive, than the RDC. Melancholia requires that *both* unreactive mood and pervasive anhedonia are present, as well as at least three additional symptoms. Thus, nearly all depressions with melancholic symptom features will meet RDC for endogenous features, but the converse is not true.

Are there therapeutic implications for the endogenous/nonendogenous dichotomy? Most evidence from the sleep laboratory and from neuroendocrine studies suggest that endogenous depressions are more likely to be associated with a higher incidence of dexamethasone nonsuppression (ie, abnormalities in hypothalamic-pituitary-adrenal axis) and with shortened REM latencies, reductions in stage 4 time, and other sleep EEG disturbances. In addition, significant correlations between antidepressant plasma levels and treatment response have been found in the endogenous but not in the nonendogenous subgroups [8]. Many believe that depressions with endogenous symptom features are more uniformly and thoroughly responsive to the antidepressant medications compared with nonendogenous depressions.

A formerly held belief that endogenous depressions occurred in normal personalities whereas nonendogenous depressions occurred in neurotic personalities appears invalid. A number of patients with endogenous depression may also suffer from disturbed, neurotic personality structures; neurotic personality does not prevent endogenous depressions, and the presence of a neurotic personality does not imply de facto that antidepressant medication will be ineffective [9,10].

Table 3.   With Melancholia

A.   Loss of pleasure in all or almost all activities

B.   Lack of reactivity to usually pleasurable stimuli

C.   At least three of the following:
   1. Distinct quality to mood
   2. Morning worsening
   3. Terminal insomnia
   4. Marked psychomotor retardation
   5. Significant anorexia/weight loss
   6. Excessive guilt

Questions that remain about this dichotomy are: (1) Are these two entities etiologically distinct? (2) Does the history of depression in first-degree relatives differentiate endogenous from nonendogenous depressions? (3) Do patients who suffer one endogenous episode display endogenous symptom features in all subsequent episodes? (4) Is the nonendogenous group more likely to benefit from re-educative psychotherapy than from medication? Currently, clinical and research evidence suggests that patients with endogenous or melancholic features respond optimally to somatic treatments. If a trial of antidepressant medication fails, the clinician should either choose another antidepressant medication or electroconvulsive therapy. In such cases, the initial focus of psychotherapy should be to provide patients with an understanding of the nature of depression and to obtain compliance with treatment. Character change, exploration of childhood experience, and focus on the "secondary gains" of the illness or the patient's "need to suffer" are not

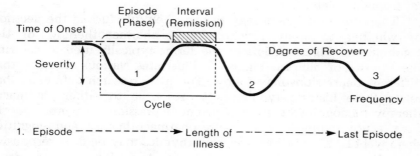

Figure 2.   Parameters course of depressions.

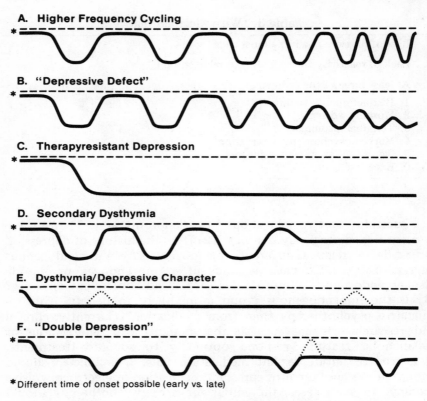

A. Higher Frequency Cycling

B. "Depressive Defect"

C. Therapyresistant Depression

D. Secondary Dysthymia

E. Dysthymia/Depressive Character

F. "Double Depression"

*Different time of onset possible (early vs. late)

Figure 3. Typology: course of depressive disorders (unipolar).

indicated and may even be counter-therapeutic, in my opinion. However, research data to support this clinical impression is presently far from complete.

The course of illness may provide helpful clues in the decision of whether to apply psychotherapy, pharmacotherapy, or the combination. Figure 2 defines the terms typically used to describe the course of illness. Figure 3 illustrates various courses that different depressions may follow. Too little research data exist that relate these historic typologies to response to either pharmacotherapy or cognitive therapy. Chronic depressions fare more poorly than acute depressions to both pharmacotherapy and cognitive therapy [11,12]. Further, some dysthymics may be drug-responsive [13]. From my clinical experience, Types A and D may be most drug-responsive. Type C may require electroconvulsive-therapy or unusual combinations of pharmacotherapy. Further, Type Cs extended period in depression may lead to more long-lasting cognitive distortions and demoralization, for which cognitive therapy may be especially helpful. Those with partial interepisode recovery (Types B and F) may also benefit from cognitive therapy. Again, these judgments are simply one clinician's suggestions; these conclusions are not based upon research data. More research into whether the course of illness has treatment implications is clearly needed.

COGNITIVE THEORY OF DEPRESSION

The cognitive theory of depression [14] is a formulation that grew out of careful clinical observation and experimental testing. This interplay of clinical and experimental information has fostered the careful evolution of this model and of the psychotherapy it has spawned. The cognitive model postulates three specific notions to explain depression: the *cognitive triad, schemas,* and *cognitive errors.* The cognitive triad consists of three major cognitive patterns that are evident in the patient's view of himself, his future, and his day-to-day experiences (world). The first component, negative view of the self, is apparent as depressed patients see themselves as defective, inadequate, or unworthy. They attribute their unpleasant experiences to physical, mental, or moral defects in themselves. Patients believe they are undesirable and worthless *because* of their presumed defects. They underestimate or criticize themselves because of these defects. Finally, they believe they lack the attributes they think are essential to the attainment of happiness and contentment. Secondly, depressed persons interpret their ongoing experiences in negative ways. They see the world as making exorbitant demands on them and/or presenting insurmountable obstacles to their reaching their life goals. They misinterpret their interactions with those around them as evidence for defeat and deprivation. These negative misinterpretations are evident in observations of depressed patients, who negatively construe situations even when less negative, more plausible alternative interpretations are available. Depressed persons realize that their initial negative interpretations are biased if they are persuaded to reflect on less negative alternative explanations. In this way, they come to realize that they tailor facts to fit their preconceived negative conclusions.

The third component, negative view of the future, is evident as depressed persons look ahead. They anticipate that current difficulties or suffering will continue indefinitely. They expect unremitting hardship, frustration, and deprivation. When they think of undertaking specific tasks, they expect to fail.

Cognitive theory considers that many associated signs and symptoms of depression are maintained or may follow from the activation of negative thinking patterns. For example, if patients incorrectly *think* they are being rejected, they react with the same negative affect (eg, sadness, anger) that occurs with *actual* rejection. If they erroneously believe they are social outcasts, they will feel lonely.

The motivational symptoms (eg, paralysis of will, escape and avoidance wishes, etc) may also be fueled by negative thinking. "Paralysis of will" may result from patients' pessimism and hopelessness. If they expect a negative outcome, they won't commit themselves to a goal or specific undertaking. Suicidal wishes are understood as extreme expressions of desires to escape from what *appears* to be insoluable problems or unbearable situations. Depressed persons often see themselves as worthless burdens and consequently believe that everyone, themselves included, are better off dead.

Increased dependency can also be explained by a cognitive perspective. Because he/she sees himself as inept and undesirable, the depressed person unrealistically overestimates the difficulty of normal tasks and expects things to turn out badly. The patient seeks help and reassurance from others whom he considers more competent and capable.

Finally, cognitive distortions may also exacerbate the physical symptoms of depression. Apathy and low energy may result from the patient's belief that he is doomed to failure in all his efforts. A negative view of the future (a sense of futility) may exacerbate "psychomotor inhibition."

Schemas

The notion of schemas is the second major ingredient in the cognitive model. Schemas explain why depressed patients cling to painful attitudes despite objective evidence of positive factors in their lives.

Any situation is composed of a plethora of stimuli. An individual selectively attends to specific stimuli, combines them into a pattern, and conceptualizes the situation. Although different persons may

Table 4. Cognitive Theory (Beck)

A. Cognitions

1. Consist of thoughts and images
2. Reflect unrealistically negative views of self, world, and future
3. Based on schemas
4. Reinforced by current interpretations of events
5. Explain symptom of depressive syndrome
6. Covary with severity of depression
7. Logical errors occur in cognitions that are negatively distorted

B. Schemas (silent assumptions)

1. Consist of unspoken, inflexible assumptions or beliefs
2. Result from past (early) experience
3. Form basis for screening, discriminating, weighting, and encoding stimuli
4. Form basis for categorizing, evaluating experiences and making judgments, and distorting actual experience
5. Determine the content of cognitions formed in situations and the affective response to them
6. Increase vulnerability to relapse

conceptualize the same situation in different ways, a particular person tends to be consistent in his responses to similar types of events. Relatively stable cognitive patterns form the basis for the regularity of interpretations of a particular set of situations.

The term "schema" designates these stable cognitive patterns. When a person faces a particular circumstance, a schema related to the circumstance is activated. The schema is the basis for molding data into cognitions (defined as any mental activity with verbal or pictorial content). A schema constitutes the basis for screening out, differentiating, and coding the stimuli that confront the individual. He/she categorizes and evaluates his/her experiences through a matrix of schemas. Schemas are inferred constructs, while cognitions are available to the persons consciousness.

The kinds of schemas employed determine how an individual will structure different experiences. A schema may be inactive at one time but can be activated by specific environmental inputs. The schemas activated in a specific situation directly determine how the person affectively responds to the circumstance. For example, if a person is concerned over whether or not he is competent and adequate, he may be assuming the validity of the schema, "Unless I do everything perfectly, I'm a failure." In this case, he will be construing situations in terms of the question of adequacy even when the question is not related to the situation. For instance, while swimming at the beach (an apparently fun activity *not* related to personal competence), this person may be thinking, "Is my swimming good enough? Do I look as good as the others?" and so forth.

Thus, the depressed patient's conceptualizations of specific situations are distorted to fit the schemas. The orderly matching of stimulus and appropriate schema is upset by the intrusion of overly active, idiosyncratic schemas that displace more appropriate ones. As these idiosyncratic schemas become more active, they are evoked by a wider range of stimuli that are less logically related to them. The patient loses control of his thinking processes and is unable to invoke other more appropriate schemas.

In milder depression, the patient is able to view his negative thoughts with some objectivity. As the depression worsens, his thinking is increasingly dominated by negative ideas, although there may be no logical connection between actual situations and negative interpretations. The patient is less able to entertain the notion that his negative interpretations are erroneous, possibly because the stronger idiosyncratic schemas interfere with reality testing and reasoning. The hypervalent schemas lead to distortions of reality and consequently to systematic errors in the depressed person's thinking.

Cognitive Errors

These systematic errors in the logic of the depressed person's thinking include arbitrary inference, selective abstraction, overgeneralization, magnification or minimization, and personalization.

1. *Arbitrary inference* refers to the process of drawings a conclusion in the absence of evidence to support the conclusion or when the evidence is contrary to the conclusion.

2. *Selective abstraction* consists of focusing on a detail taken out of context, ignoring other more salient features of the situation, and conceptualizing the whole experience on the basis of this element.

3. *Overgeneralization* refers to the pattern of drawing a general conclusion on the basis of a single incident.

4. *Magnification and minimization* is reflected in errors in evaluation that are so gross as to constitute a distortion.

5. *Personalization* refers to the patient's proclivity to relate external events to himself when there is no basis of making such a connection.

Cognitive theory offers a hypothesis about the predisposition to depression. Briefly, the notion is that early experiences constitute a basis for forming a negative view about one's self, the future, and the world around. Schemas may be latent, but they can be activated by specific circumstances which are analogous to experiences initially responsible for embedding the negative attitude.

For example, disruption of a marital situation may activate the concept of irreversible loss associated with death of a parent in childhood. Alternatively, depression may be triggered by a physical abnormality or disease that activates the notion that he is destined for a life of suffering. While these and other events might be painful to most people, they would not necessarily produce a depression unless the person is particularly sensitive to the situation because of previous experience and consequent predepressive cognitive organization.

In response to such traumas, the average person will still maintain interest in and realistically appraise other nontraumatic aspects of his life. However, the thinking of the depression-prone person becomes markedly constricted and negative ideas develop about every aspect of his life.

There is substantial empirical support for the cognitive theory of depression from naturalistic studies, clinical observations, and experimental studies [15,16]. Studies have documented the presence and intercorrelation of the constituents of the "cognitive triad" in association with depression. Several studies document the presence of specific cognitive deficits (eg, impaired abstract reasoning, selective attention) in depressed or suicidal persons. The presence of dysfunctional attitudes or schemas has been found with depressed patients. Although more experimental investigations are needed, cognitive theory has led to a specific psychotherapy for depression and other forms of psychopathology [17].

AN OVERVIEW OF THE PROCEDURE OF COGNITIVE THERAPY

Cognitive theory forms the basis for cognitive therapeutic methods. The therapy consists of a number of specific techniques for treating depressed patients, as well as a theoretical perspective by which to organize the clinical data, to conceptualize the treatment plan, and to proceed in the conduct of therapy. These techniques and procedures have been detailed elsewhere [1]. This section will illustrate a few of these techniques to provide a flavor for how treatment is conducted.

Cognitive therapy is a short-term, time-limited psychotherapy usually involving a maximum of 20 sessions over 10 to 12 weeks. The therapist actively directs the discussion to focus on selected problem areas or target symptoms presented by the patient. Questioning is frequently used to elicit specific thoughts, images, definitions, and meanings. For example, the therapist might say, "What did the phone call mean to you?", or "What were you thinking just as you hung up the telephone?" In addition, questioning is used to expose inner contradictions, inconsistencies, and logical flaws in the patient's thinking or conclusions. Skill and tact are required, however, to assure that this questioning is not construed as an interrogation or cross-examination by patients. Such a view might lead the depressed person to conclude that his reasoning powers are defective.

The therapist and patient collaborate in the use of empirical methodology to focus on specific problem areas. The therapist must clearly understand the patient's conceptualizations of himself and the world around him. In essence, he must be able to see the world "through the patient's eyes." If the patient's conceptualizations differ from the therapist's view of reality, the collaborators tend to reconcile the differences with a logical-empirical approach.

In essence, the patient's thoughts are treated as if they were hypotheses requiring validation. During this validation process (often conducted as homework), the patient needs to clearly understand what beliefs or ideas (hypotheses) are being tested and, therefore, must understand the purpose of each homework assignment. Technically, cognitive therapy may be compared with a scientific investigation: (1) collecting data that are as reliable and valid as possible, (2) formulating hypotheses based on these data, and (3) testing and, if indicated, revising the hypotheses or thinking patterns based on new information.

The data consist of the patient's "automatic thoughts" or cognitions. These automatic thoughts are collected as oral or written reports from the patient. The therapist accepts these thoughts as truthful (although not necessarily *accurate*) representations of reality, since a basic premise of cognitive theory is that the depressed person negatively misconstrues his experiences.

First, the therapist tries to elicit automatic thoughts surrounding each upsetting event. He tries to obtain specific evidence for or against the patient's potentially distorted or dysfunctional thinking by questioning the patient about the total circumstance of a particular event.

Secondly, the cognitive therapist helps the patient to identify or infer the assumptions or attitudes that underpin the recurrent negative automatic thinking. For example, such a theme might be "expecting to fail" or "reading rejection into personal situations." The therapist helps the patient to see that such beliefs may not necessarily reflect reality. For example, the therapist would use logic, persuasion, and evidence from the patient's current and past functioning to get the patient to view a belief (eg, "I am unable to learn") as an idea or hypothesis requiring validation, rather than as a belief.

Thirdly, the cognitive therapist teaches the patient to identify specific errors of logic in his thinking (eg, arbitrary inference, over-generalization, etc). Learning to recognize and correct these errors helps the patient to repeatedly assess the degree to which his thinking mirrors reality.

The patient and therapist collaborate to identify basic attitudes, beliefs, and assumptions, which (according to the model) shape moment-to-moment thinking. Sometimes, an attitude may be so dominant or pervasive that despite changes in environmental events, the conclusion never varies (eg, "I can't be happy unless I'm loved"). By articulating these attitudes, the therapist helps the patient not only to develop a basis for empirical validation, but also to recognize subsequent cognitions based on these attitudes.

Cognitive therapy techniques are designed to facilitate changes in specific target symptoms found in depression (eg, inactivity, self-criticism, lack of gratification, suicidal wishes). In general, a therapy session begins with a discussion of the previously assigned homework. This homework generally focuses on the patient's thinking. The latter part of each session is spent developing and planning the next homework assignment.

In the initial sessions, therapy tends to emphasize increased activity and environmental interaction (ie, behavioral changes). In the course of such changes, the patient learns to recognize and record the thinking associated with particular behaviors, activities, or changes in mood. This early emphasis on behavioral objectives is based on our recognition that the severely depressed patient is often unable to engage in cognitive tasks because of difficulty in abstract reasoning.

As the depression lessens, concentration improves and the intensity of the affect decreases. The patient is taught to collect, examine, and empirically test his negative automatic thinking. In subsequent sessions, the assumptions supporting the cognitions are identified and subjected to empirical validation through homework assignments. These cognitive-change techniques require a greater ability to abstract and use logic. Therefore, they are employed after the depression lessens in severity. However, the therapist may employ these cognitive change techniques from the outset if the patient is only moderately depressed. In addition, a task designed mainly to alter behavior, will also influence the patient's thinking. Similarly, a cognitive change may result in a behavioral change as well.

Table 5 lists several behaviorally oriented techniques, and Table 6 lists some techniques aimed more particularly at changing cognitions or beliefs. These lists of techniques are not exhaustive [1]. In fact, an experienced cognitive therapist will design homework assignments for each individual patient in each session depending on the cognitive and behavioral targets to be addressed.

Homework assignments are critical to treatment. They are designed to help patients: (1) develop objectivity about situations that otherwise are stereotypically misconstrued, (2) idenfity underlying assumptions, and (3) develop and test alternative conceptualizations and guiding assumptions.

The therapist selects specific techniques depending upon the degree and type of psychotherapy present [1,18]. For example, the therapist provides greater structure, direction, and guidance to more severely depressed patients who are less able to think objectively. Typically, therapy begins with techniques that focus on behavioral monitoring and change. These techniques are often very simple. They are designed to provide patients with success experiences. Subsequently, task assignments are given to provide stimuli for the collection and later correction of cognitions.

With few exceptions [19,20], there is not much empirical evidence as yet to document the efficacy of this approach, except

Table 5. Behavioral Techniques

Activity scheduling
Mastery and pleasure ratings
Graded task assignment
Cognitive rehearsal
Assertive training/role playing
Mood graph

Table 6.   Cognitive Techniques

Recording automatic thoughts (cognitions)
Reattribution techniques
Responding to negative cognitions
Counting automatic thoughts
Identifying assumptions
Modifying shoulds
Pro-con refutation of assumptions
Homework to test old assumptions
Homework to test new assumptions

in depression. The available outcome studies in depression suggest that patients who are particularly suitable for this approach suffer from mild-moderate unipolar, nonpsychotic depression, and they have the capacity to establish a working alliance in a short period of time. These patients appear most likely to obtain significant symptom reduction in ten weeks of treatment. Chronic depressions are *not* more responsive and may be less responsive than more acute disorders [21]. Depressions with melancholic features [2] have not been systematically evaluated. At this point, such patients should receive chemotherapy or electroconvulsive therapy as a primary treatment.

It is controversial as to whether those patients with endogenous features according to Research Diagnostic Criteria [7] will respond to cognitive therapy [22,23]. While the answer to this question awaits further research, the clinician is well advised *not* to utilize cognitive therapy alone in such patients in order to obtain symptom reduction. On the other hand, recall that symptom reduction is *not* the only objective of cognitive or other psychotherapies. While evidence for the prophylactic effect of cognitive therapy is scanty, it is conceivable that some patients may reach a better level of interepisode recovery because of cognitive therapy even if anti-depressant medications are essential for initially obtaining symptom reduction.

For example, consider a patient who has endured three episodes of major depression with substantial but not total interepisode recovery. Assume further that the patient has obtained a near full symptomatic remission with amitriptyline. The patient has still experienced a good deal of time in the recent past in the depressed state. Might this experience not have affected his view of himself, his sense of competence, and his view of things around him? Pharmacotherapy may not be as effective as cognitive psychotherapy in modifying such views, at least in the short run [24,25]. Such a patient might profit from a short course (five to ten weeks) of cognitive therapy to help him become more objective about both himself and his illness.

Thus, cognitive therapy may be indicated in a patient who requires antidepressants for symptom reduction and/or prophylaxis, but who also needs to relearn or unlearn specific self-defeating views or notions that either preceded or arose in conjunction with the symptomatic manifestation of the depression.

CONTRAINDICATIONS

While Beck et al [1] caution that many depressed patients may require medication or may not respond to cognitive therapy, specific *contraindications* to this treatment are yet to be identified. Clinical experience suggests that patients with impaired reality testing (eg, hallucinations, delusions), impaired reasoning abilities or memory function (eg, organic brain syndromes), borderline personality structures, and schizoaffective disorder will not respond to this treatment, at least in its short-term format [1,17,18]. Whether antisocial personalities with major depression or other forms of secondary depressions will respond to cognitive therapy is yet to be empirically established. However, clinical experience suggests that many secondary depressions will respond.

The clinical experience of several cognitive therapists suggests that major depressions that accompany medical disorders, but *are not biologically caused* by such disorders (ie, *not* Organic Affective Disorders by DSM-III), may respond rapidly to cognitive therapy, especially in patients who do not have a history of preexisting psychopathology. For example, patients with their first myocardial infarction, with some forms of cancer, and/or with physical injuries that require substantial psychological readjustment (eg, blindness, loss of limb) can profit from this approach in very short order (eg, five weeks). Those with more chronic, disabling, and progressive medical illnesses may profit to some degree, but respond more slowly.

The reasons for failure with cognitive therapy have been the subject of a recent review [26]. One possible contraindication has been suggested based on a subtype of depression, namely, endogenous depression with associated dexamethasone nonsuppression [27–29]. Five patients with severe endogenous depressions and dexamethasone nonsuppression who were treated by the author all failed to respond at all to cognitive therapy alone. However, such recommendations are as yet based on anecdotal information. Perhaps in the future, specific biological measures will help to identify responders and non-responders to cognitive or other psychotherapies.

Most patients who ultimately respond well in terms of acute symptom reduction will do so within five to seven weeks of twice-a-week treatment with cognitive therapy alone. If 50 percent symptom reduction by Hamilton Rating Scale [30] or Beck Depression Inventory [31] is *not* achieved by 14 sessions, the treatment plan should be revised.

It is suprising that there are as yet no reports of adverse reactions to cognitive therapy. Adverse reactions may be difficult to differentiate from lack of efficacy. For instance, suicide attempts, as well as premature terminations, may be evidence of either adverse reactions or lack of efficacy. Two studies [32,33] found that cognitive behavioral methods were associated with a significantly lower premature dropout rate than antidepressant pharmacotherapy alone, while a more recent report [11] did not replicate these findings. One might suspect that the structured, planned, directive nature of this approach helps retain depressed outpatients in treatment. If so, cognitive therapy might be particularly useful in outpatients of lower socioeconomic class, whose dropout rate from psychotherapy is particularly high [34].

COMBINING COGNITIVE THERAPY AND PHARMACOTHERAPY IN DEPRESSION

In terms of overall objectives, both pharmacotherapy and short-term psychotherapies aim at reduction or removal of symptoms ("secondary prevention"), the prevention of relapse (prophylaxis), and/or the reduction of the secondary consequences of the disorder ("tertiary" prevention). While various psychotherapies may share these common overall objectives, the intermediate objectives or steps used to obtain symptom reduction or prophylaxis may distinguish specific psychotherapies. Furthermore, psychotherapy may be useful to increase adherence to medication prescription.

Psychotherapy may be directed at specific symptoms or problem behaviors; for example, relaxation and desensitization are used in phobic conditions. Alternatively, therapy may focus on the patient's interaction with his/her social system. Therapy may address psychological processes, identified within the individual patient or members of the social system, that are presumed to produce, maintain, or exacerbate symptomatology or to predispose to relapse or to secondary disability.

Questions regarding when to combine the use of psychotherapy and chemotherapy are even more complicated and, as yet, not well-answered by empirical data. For which patients or which disorders are both treatments indicated? Does each treatment accomplish a different goal? How do the two approaches interact? Are certain types of psychotherapy more compatible with pharmacotherapy, while others are antagonistic to it? When in the course of an illness is psychotherapy actually indicated?

The therapeutic effects of pharmacotherapy depend upon a variety of factors. A few of these factors are the chemical effects of the specific agent, the dosage employed, the length of time the drug is prescribed, patient adherence to the regime, and the disorder under treatment. Similarly, if "psychotherapy" has specific therapeutic effects, it would be logical to expect that these effects will depend on the psychological effects of the treatment, the length of the treatment and the frequency of the sessions, the patient's participation in therapy, and the disorder under treatment. Only recently have the latter speculations begun to receive support from empirical research.

Cognitive therapy has been most thoroughly assessed in non-psychotic, nonbipolar depressed outpatients. While many studies have been conducted on "depressed college student volunteers," several recent trials have been carried out on psychiatric patients. In one study [33], cognitive therapy exceeded the effects of imipramine. Three more recent studies also contrasted behavioral-cognitive therapy, or Beck's cognitive therapy, with antidepressant medication. McLean and Hasktian [32] reported that the behavioral-cognitive approach exceeded the effects of amitriptyline (150 mg/day). In addition, it exceeded the effects of relaxation training and short-term dynamic psychotherapy. Blackburn and coworkers [11,23] found that in depressed outpatients treated in general practice, Beck's cognitive therapy exceeded the effects of antidepressant medication. On the other hand, in psychiatric clinic outpatients, cognitive therapy equalled the effects of antidepressant medication. However, by several outcome measures, the combination treatment (cognitive therapy plus antidepressant medication) exceeded either treatment alone in this group. In a near replication of the Rush et al [33], study Murphy and coworkers [34] found that cognitive therapy equalled the effects of nortriptyline alone and of the combination of both, as well as the effect obtained by active placebo plus cognitive therapy. Only one study [35] has evaluated the question of whether the format (eg, group versus individual) affects the efficacy of cognitive therapy. The group format appeared to be *less* effective than individual therapy. A couples format has not been formally studied, although cognitive therapy can be easily adapted to this format. One clinical report [36] has suggested specific indications and techniques for involving the couple in cognitive therapy of depression. More studies are needed to evaluate the relationship of format to outcome.

The question of when and whether to combine antidepressant medication with psychotherapy remains unanswered [1,28]. Three reports have evaluated the combination of cognitive therapy with medication. Rush and Watkins [34], in a small study, found no difference between individual cognitive therapy alone and the combination of cognitive therapy plus antidepressant indications in outpatients. However, the sample size may have precluded detection of significant differences. Recently, Beck et al [1] found that adding amitriptyline did not add to the efficacy of cognitive therapy alone. Other evidence [11] indicates that with depressed outpatients treated in general practice, cognitive therapy alone was equivalent to the combination treatment; with psychiatric clinic outpatients, however, the combination treatment exceeded cognitive therapy alone. This study suggests that patient source may influence the probability of response to combination treatment. Murphy et al [34] did not find that the combination exceeded the effects obtained with either cognitive therapy alone or with medication alone. Apparently some, but clearly not all, patients are uniquely benefited by the combination treatment. Other patients may benefit from cognitive therapy without medication.

CAUSES OF FAILURE WITH COGNITIVE THERAPY

Treatment failures are perhaps the most instructive of all experiences for psychotherapists. The lessons gleaned from each failure have implications for improved patient selection, refinements and innovations in psychotherapeutic techniques, differential diagnosis of the disorders themselves (ie, some types of depression may be unresponsive to psychotherapy), improving compliance with homework, improving strategies to deal with counter-therapeutic social system forces, and identification of patients who have only short-term as opposed to long-term gains.

Perhaps the most commonly offered rationale for treatment failures in general is "the patient isn't motivated." There is an especially great temptation to attribute "lack of motivation" to those depressed patients who fail to respond. However, this "explanation" is, in fact, both logically untenable and obfuscating. Depression, the syndrome [2], involves by definition a reduction in energy and motivation. Thus, all depressed patients are less motivated than normal subjects to undertake most activities, including psychotherapy. In cognitive therapy, the patient is required both to attend the sessions and to complete various homework assignments in order to obtain a therapeutic effect. These requirements are being leveled at patients, all of whom are "unmotivated." Thus, "lack of motivation" explains all failures. However, those who do respond are also "unmotivated" at the outset. Therefore, lack of motivation is associated with both successes and failures (ie, it explains nothing).

There are, of course, some patients who appear more or less difficult to engage in the treatment process. We believe this initial differential tendency to collaborate evolves out of two major forces: difficulty with trust and the pervasiveness and certainty of the negative anticipations held by the patient. Each of these issues, trust and negative anticipations, are reframed in cognitive terms and dealt with very early in treatment. Negative anticipations are elicited by the therapist and corrected with information, logical discussion, and experimental tasks [1]. Trust issues are also reframed in cognitive terms. For example, the patient may believe, "If I really tell you (the therapist) how I think, you won't like me." There is often an anticipation of rejection or disappointment underlying the patient's reluctance to engage as a full collaborator with the therapist. Such patients will often begin to work in treatment and then back off, reduce compliance, and voice more hopeless and helpless notions. These notions not atypically also involve denigration of the therapist or the therapy process. Such behaviors and views may serve to protect the patient from developing an emotional, personal relationship (a therapeutic alliance) and, consequently, avoid the presumed rejection and disappointment as the treatment is terminated. Again, these fears are identified, framed cognitively into "if . . . , then . . ." statements (eg, "If I put my hopes into this treatment or the therapist and don't get better, I'll be shattered or it means I'm incurable, etc . . .") and discussed logically.

More severely depressed patients are especially likely to suffer from difficulties in trust and severe negative anticipation of the future. As such, the engagement of these patients is both critical and difficult [18]. However, by first identifying behavioral patterns that appear to represent these assumptions, by raising these assumptions in the form of questions early in treatment, and by addressing them repeatedly throughout treatment, the therapist can usually engage such "unmotivated" patients.

Aside from general intelligence, which we do not feel is a critical factor in dictating success or failure, there are a number of clinical situations that can lead to failure. These include impairments in memory or concentration found in either severe depressions or early organic brain syndrome. Patients with the latter are especially likely to seek help because of low energy, sleep difficulties, sadness or apathy, and a reduced sense of self-esteem. Careful medical and psychiatric evaluation can exclude patients with these disorders.

In addition, patients will often present with minor or even major depressions [2] that are consequences of some underlying un-diagnosed medical disorder or medication. Our experience at South-western Medical School, Affective Disorders Clinic, is that 15 to 20 percent of "depressed" outpatients have such disorders. Cognitive therapy will not work in these cases.

One 35-year-old woman with sadness, insomnia, self-criticism, low energy, poor concentration, weight and appetite reductions, and headaches was evaluated by both a psychiatrist and psychologist before agreeing to and participating in cognitive therapy. After 20 sessions, her self-critical attitudes, according to the patient, were reduced. However, she stated, "I'm still depressed," and indeed her other symptoms were basically unchanged. A reevaluation was conducted. It was discovered that she had been taking alpha-methyldopa, an antihypertensive agent, that can cause depression. She had previously reported that she was taking no medications because "I've been taking these blood pressure pills for years." Her depressive symptoms disappeared completely within three weeks after the medication was stopped.

The second case, 34-year-old nurse with multiple sclerosis that resulted in mild disabilities in motor coordination that did not preclude her continued full-time employment, developed a major depressive episode [2]. She complained of apathy, loss of interest and pleasure, insomnia, low energy, suicidal thinking, and mild reductions in weight and appetite. She was chiefly preoccupied with anticipations of massive disability as her multiple sclerosis progressed. These thoughts were clearly negatively biased in that her actual disabilities were relatively mild and her illness was in relatively good control.

After 20 sessions of cognitive therapy, no relief of any of her symptoms ensued. She was then tried on two different tricyclic antidepressant medications, both of which failed. She was admitted to the hospital, where a thorough medical, neurological, and laboratory evaluation revealed severe hypothyroidism. Treatment with thyroid replacement completely relieved all of her symptoms including her negatively biased thinking. She returned to work and has remained asymptomatic for two years.

The latter case illustrates the presence of two seperate medical disorders, one of which caused the depression. The therapist had initially felt that "anyone with multiple sclerosis would be depressed" and erroneously attributed her depressive symptoms to the stress of her neurological disease. If that diagnosis were correct, then symptomatic response should have followed cognitive therapy. Thus, a failure to respond to cognitive therapy should lead the clinician to completely reevaluate the case. In addition, a thorough medical and psychiatric evaluation *before* beginning cognitive or behavioral treatment for depression is essential, even if the patient "knows why" he or she is depressed. Medications and medical illnesses produce mood changes and other symptoms of the depressive syndrome, including cognitive symptoms sych as negative views of the self, world, and future, Consequently, psychologically minded patients with an unrecognized medical illness that causes depressive symptoms can often provide themselves and the therapist with a convincing but invalid story as to why they are depressed.

A final major deterrent to therapeutic effect may consist of forces within the patient's social system. Significant others may unwittingly conceptualize the depressed patient as a helpless, negative, hostile person from whom nothing better can be anticipated in the future. This situation is most likely to ensue when the depression has been present for a longer period of time. Many depressed patients will overvalue the opinions and views of others. Thus, in the course of cognitive therapy, behavioral or attitudinal changes hoped for by the therapist and practiced by the patient may be undercut by the fixed views of the patient held by significant others.

Several therapeutic strategies have been suggested in anecdotal reports [1,36]. Basically, if such counter-therapeutic social forces exist, it is imperative that the couple or family system members be engaged in the process of cognitive change. Often, these negative significant others have themselves lost hope of seeing meaningful changes in the index patient. Behaviors and attitudes generated by the depression, are attributed, erroneously, to the patient's character. Significant others can be employed to therapeutic benefit as assistants in obtaining compliance with homework, in practicing alternative views themselves of the patient's behaviors, and in modifying the reinforcement contingencies available to the patient under the therapist's direction.

CONCLUSIONS

The efficacy of cognitive therapy in depressed, nonbipolar, nonpsychotic outpatients is suggested by virtually all studies conducted to date. On the other hand, it is clearly not effective in all patients. A similar statement may be made for antidepressant medication. The data available do not uniformly support the notion that the combined treatment always improves the symptom reduction obtained by either treatment alone. The empirical evidence available does not help us readily determine for which individual the use of either drugs, cognitive therapy, or the combination is indicated. My clinical impression (not yet tested rigorously) is that most non-endogenous depressions will fare well with cognitive therapy alone, whereas many endogenous depressions will respond completely to pharmacotherapy alone. When interepisode recovery is partial, when many months or years have been spent in depression which may teach patients to think negatively even when not fully depressed, or when social system forces prevent revisions in self-concept, cognitive therapy may have a place in combination with medication. Hopefully, subsequent research will clarify the indications and contra-indications for each treatment alone and for the combination.

REFERENCES

1. Beck AT, Rush AJ, Shaw BF, Emery G: *Cognitive Therapy of Depression*. New York: Guilford Press, 1979
2. American Psychiatric Association: Diagnostic and Statistical Manual for Mental Disorders, 3rd ed. Washington, DC, 1980

3. van Praag HM, Uleman AM, Spitz JC: The vital syndrome interview: a structured standard interview for the recognition and registration of the vital depressive syndrome complex. *Psychiat Neurol Neurochir* 68:329–346, 1965
4. Rush AJ, Altshuler KZ: *Recent Advances in Diagnosis and Treatment of Depression.* New York: Guilford Press, in press
5. Lloyd C: Life events and depressive disorders reviewed. *Arch Gen Psychiatry* 37:541–548, 1980
6. Paykel ES: Contribution of life events to causation of psychiatric illness. *Psychol Med* 8:245–253, 1978
7. Spitzer RL, Endicott J, Robins E: Research diagnostic criteria: rationale and reliability. *Arch Gen Psychiatry* 3:773–782, 1978
8. Reisby N, Graham LE, Bech P, et al: Imipramine: clinical effects and pharmacokinetic variability. *Psychopharmacology* 54:263–272, 1977
9. van Praag HM: A transatlantic view of the diagnosis of depression according to DSM-III: I. Controversies and misunderstandings in depression diagnosis. *Compr Psychiatry* 23:315–329, 1982a
10. van Praag HM: A transatlantic view of the diagnosis of depression according to DSM-III: II. Did the DSM-III solve the problem of depression diagnosis? *Compr Psychiatry* 23:3310–3338, 1982b
11. Blackburn I, Bishop S, Glen AIM, Whalley LJ, Christie JE, The efficacy of cognitive therapy in depression. A trial treatment using cognitive therapy and pharmacotherapy, each alone and in combination. *Br Psychiatry* 139:181–189, 1981
12. Rush AJ, Hollen SD, Beck AT, Kovacs M: Depression: must pharmacotherapy fail for cognitive therapy to succeed? *Cog Ther Res* 2:199–206, 1978
13. Akiskal HS: Dysthymic disorder: Psychopathology of proposed chronic depressive subtypes. *Am J Psychiatry* 140:11–20, 1983
14. Beck AT: *Cognitive Therapy and The Emotional Disorders.* New York: International Universities Press, 1976
15. Beck AT, Rush AJ: Cognitive approaches to depression and suicide. In *Cognitive Defects in Development of Mental Illnesss.* Edited by Serban G. New York: Brunner/Mazel, 1978
16. Giles DE, Rush AJ: Relationship of dysfunctional attitudes and dexamethasone response in endogenous and nonendogenous depression. *Biol Psychiatry* 17:1303–1314, 1982
17. Rush AJ (ed): *Short-Term Psychotherapies for Depression.* New York: Guilford Press, 1982
18. Rush AJ: Psychotherapy of the affective psychoses. *Am J Psychoanal* 40:99–123, 1980
19. Khatami M, Rush AJ: A pilot study of the treatment of outpatients with chronic pain: symptom control, stimulus control, and social system intervention. *Pain* 5:163–172, 1978
20. Khatami M, Rush AJ: One year followup of multimodal treatment of chronic pain, in press
21. Rush AJ, Hollon S, Beck AT, Kovacs M: Depression: must pharmacotherapy fail for cognitive therapy to succeed? *Cog Ther Res* 2:199–206, 1978
22. Kovacs M, Rush AJ, Beck AT, Hollon SD: Depressed outpatient treated with cognitive therapy or pharmacotherapy. A one-year followup. *Arch Gen Psychiatry* 38:33–39, 1981

23. Blackburn I, Bishop S: Is there an alternative to drugs in the treatment of depressed ambulatory patients? *Behav Psychother* 9:96-104, 1981

24. Rush AJ, Beck AT, Kovacs M, Weissenburger J, Hollon S: Differential effects of cognitive therapy and pharmacotherapy on hopelessness and self concept. *Am J Psychiatry* 139:862-866, 1982

25. Rush AJ, Giles DE, Roffwarg HP, Parker CR: Sleep EEG dexamethasone suppression test findings in outpatients with unipolar major depressive disorders. *Biol Psychiatry* 17:327-341, 1982

26. Rush AJ, Shaw BF: Failure in treating depression by cognitive behavioral therapy. In *Failures in Behavior Therapy*, edited by Emmelkamp PM, Foa EB. New York: Wiley and Sons, 1983

27. Carroll BJ, Feinberg M, Greden JF, Tarika J, Albala AA, Hakett RF, James James NMcI, Kronfol Z, Lohr N, Steiner M, deVigne JP, Young E: A specific laboratory test for the diagnosis of melancholia, *Arch Gen Psychiatry* 38:15-22, 1981

28. Rush AJ: Biological markers and treatment response in affective disorders *McLean Hospital Bull* 8:38-61, 1983a

29. Rush AJ,: Clinical and etiological implications of biologic derangements in major depression. In *Affective Disorders*, edited by Maas J, Davis J. Washington, DC: American Psychiatric Press, 1983

30. Hamilton M: A rating scale for depression. *J Neurol Neurosurg Psychiatry* 12:56-62, 1960

31. Beck AT, Ward CH, Mendelson M, Mock JE, Erbaugh JK: An inventory for measuring depression *Arch Gen Psychiatry* 4:561-571, 1961

32. McLean PD, Hakstian AR: Clinical depression: comparative efficacy of outpatient treatments. *J Consult Clin Psychol* 47:818-836, 1979

33. Rush AJ, Beck AT, Kovacs M, Hollon S: Comparative efficacy of cognitive therapy and pharmacotherapy in the treatment of depressed outpatients. *Cog Ther Res* 1:17-37, 1977

34. Murphy GE, Simons AD, Wetzel RD, Lustman PJ: Cognitive therapy and antidepressant medication, individually and in combination, versus cognitive therapy plus placebo as control in the treatment of depression: treatment outcome. *Arch Gen Psychiatry* in press

35. Rush AJ, Watkins JT: Group versus individual cognitive therapy: a pilot study. *Cog Ther Res* 5:95-103, 1981

36. Rush AJ, Shaw B, Khatami M: Cognitive therapy of depression: utilizing the couples system. *Cog Ther Res* 4:103-113, 1980

CHAPTER 8

Depression: Interpersonal Psychotherapy and Tricyclics

Myrna M. Weissman and Gerald L. Klerman

A social or interpersonal approach does not deny the importance of unconscious mental process of childhood experience or of biological vulnerability or personality traits, but they reach their capacity to determine behavior through their ability to influence the patient's definition of the situation in the 'here and now.'

Harry Stack Sullivan
The Interpersonal Theory of Psychiatry
New York: W. W. Norton, 1953

INTRODUCTION

Interpersonal psychotherapy (IPT) is based on the evidence that most clinical depressions—regardless of symptom patterns, severity, presumed biological vulnerability, or personality traits—occur in an interpersonal context. Understanding and renegotiating the interpersonal context associated with the depression is important to the depressed person's recovery and in the prevention of possible further episodes. IPT is a brief (usually 12 to 16 weeks) weekly psychotherapeutic treatment developed for the ambulatory, nonbipolar, nonpsychotic depressed patient, focused on improving the quality of the depressed patient's current interpersonal functioning. It is suitable for use, after appropriate training, by experienced psychiatrists, psychologists, or social workers. It can be used alone or in conjunction with pharmacologic approaches.

IPT has evolved from the New Haven-Boston Collaborative Depression Project over 15 years of experience in the treatment and research of ambulatory depressed patients. It has been tested alone, in comparison, and in combination with tricyclics in two clinical trials with depressed patients, one of maintenance [1,2], and one of acute treatment [3,4]. Four additional clinical trials with depressed patients are currently underway [5].

The concept, techniques, and methods of IPT have been operationally described in a manual that has undergone a number of revisions [6]. This manual was developed to standardize the treatment so that clinical trials could be undertaken. A training program for experienced psychotherapists of different disciplines providing the treatment for these clinical trials has been developed.

It is our experience that a variety of treatments may be suitable for depression and that the depressed patient's interests are best served by the availability and scientific testing of different psychological as well as pharmacological treatments, to be used alone or in combination. Ultimately, clinical testing and experience will determine which is the best treatment for the particular patient.

This paper describes the theoretical and empirical basis for IPT, summarizes the procedures for conducting IPT, and presents data demonstrating its efficacy in comparison and in combination with tricyclics with ambulatory depressed patients.

Theoretical Framework for IPT

IPT is derived from a number of theoretical sources. The earliest is Adolph Meyer [7], whose psychobiological approach to understanding psychiatric disorders placed great emphasis on the patient's current psychosocial and interpersonal experiences. In contrast to Kraepelin and the concept of psychiatric illness, derived from continental European psychiatry, Meyer saw psychiatric disorders as part of the patient's attempt to adapt to the environment, usually the psychosocial environment. Meyer viewed the patient's response to environmental changes as determined by early developmental experiences, especially in the family, and by the patient's membership in various social groups. Meyer attempted to apply the Darwinian concept of adaptation to understanding psychiatric illness.

Among Meyer's associates, Sullivan [8,9] stands out for his theory on interpersonal relations and also for his writings linking clinical psychiatry to anthropology, sociology, and social psychology. The theoretical foundation of IPT was best summarized by Sullivan, who noted that psychiatry is the scientific study of people and the processes that involve or go between people, as distinct from the exclusive study of the mind, of society, or the brain.

The IPT emphasis on interpersonal and social factors in the understanding and treatment of depressive disorders draws upon the work of many others, especially Fromm-Reichmann and Cohen [10] and more recently Arieti and Bemporad [11]. Among others, Becker [12] and Chodoff [13] have also emphasized the social roots of depression and the need to attend to the interpersonal aspects of the disorder. An interpersonal conceptualization has been applied to psychotherapy in the writings of Frank [14], who stressed mastery of current interpersonal situations as an important component in psychotherapy.

THE EMPIRICAL BASIS FOR UNDERSTANDING DEPRESSION IN AN INTERPERSONAL CONTEXT

The empirical basis for understanding and treating depression in an interpersonal context derives from several divergent sources, including development research on ethological work with animals, the study of children, and clinical and epidemiologic studies of adults. This review of empirical studies is not meant to be exhaustive.

Attachment Bonds and Depression

Attachment theory has emphasized that the most intense human emotions are associated with the formation, disruption, and renewal of affectional attachment bonds. The studies of Bowlby [15], based on earlier investigations of the animal ethologists and later applied to studying the mother-child relationship, have demonstrated the importance of attachment and social bonds to human functioning, the vulnerability of individuals to impaired interpersonal relations if strong attachment bonds did not develop early, and the vulnerability of individuals to depression or despair during disruption of attachment bonds. Many types of psychiatric disorders result in a person's inability to make and keep affectional bonds. The way in which the individual forms affectional bonds is learned largely by experience within the family, especially, but not exclusively, during early childhood.

Based on these observations, Bowlby [16] proposed a rationale for psychotherapy. Psychotherapy is designed to assist the patient in examining current interpersonal relationships in order to understand how they may be construed on the basis of the patient's experiences with attachment figures in childhood, adolescence, and adulthood.

The work of Bowlby has been extended by Rutter [17] to show that relationships other than that of the mother and child have an impact on the formation of attachment bonds. Closely derived from these effects has been the work of Henderson and his colleagues [18]. In a series of studies, this group has found that deficiency in social bonds in the current environment is associated with neurotic distress. However, it is unclear whether there is a real deficiency in bonds or whether the deficiency is a reflection of the depressed person's negative cognition.

Intimacy as a Protection Against Depression

The most sophisticated empirical work defining an aspect of attachment bonding (ie, intimacy and a confiding relationship) and examining its relationship to the development of depression has been completed by Brown et al [19]. In a community survey of women living in the Camberwell section of London, this group found that the presence of an intimate, confiding relationship with a man, usually the spouse, was the most important protection against developing a depression in the face of life stress.

In similar work with medical patients, Miller and Ingham [20] found that women who reported the lack of an intimate confidant to general physicians had more severe psychological symptoms.

Recent Social Stress and the Onset of Depression

Stemming from the demonstration in 1950 by Holmes, Goodell, and Wolf [21] that the rate of upper respiratory illness increases with the number of life events, a considerable body of research demonstrating the relationship between "stress" (defined as recent life events), and the onset of psychiatric illness, particularly depression, has emerged.

The studies of Paykel et al [22] are most relevant to the study of stressful life events and depression. This group studied depressed patients and found that exits of persons from the social field occurred more frequently with depressed patients than such exits occurred with normal subjects in the six months before the onset of depression. This group also found that marital friction was the most common event reported by depressed patients before the onset of depression.

Similar observations were made by Ilfeld [23] in a survey of about 3,000 adults in Chicago. Depressive symptoms were closely related to stress, particularly to stresses in marriage but less frequently to those of parenting. In a closer look at the data, Pearlin and Lieberman [24] found that chronically persisting problems within intact marriages were as likely to produce distress and depressive symptoms as was the total disruption of the marriage by divorce or separation.

Bloom, Asher, and White [25], in a critical analysis of several studies related to the consequences of marital disputes and divorce, linked these events (marital disruption) with a wide variety of emotional disorders, including depression.

Impairment of Interpersonal Relations
Associated with Clinical Depression

The impairment in close interpersonal relations of depressed women has been studied in considerable detail by Weissman and Paykel [26]. In a comparison study of depressed women and their normal neighbors, they found that the depressed women were considerably more impaired in all aspects of social functioning—as workers, wives, mothers, family members, and friends. This impairment was greatest with close family, particularly spouses and children, with whom considerable hostility, disaffection, and poor communication were evident. With symptomatic recovery, most, but not all, of the social inpairments diminished. Marital relationships often remained chronically unhappy and explosive. There has been some debate as to whether the marital difficulties associated with depression are the cause or the consequence of the disorder [27,28]. Studying the interactions of depressed patients and normal subjects, Coyne [29] has demonstrated that depressives elicit characteristic, unhelpful responses from others.

This brief review summarizes some of the key empirical findings that provide a rationale for understanding depression in an interpersonal context and for developing a psychotherapy for depression based on interpersonal concepts. In general, studies show the importance of close and satisfactory attachments to others in the prevention of depression, and, alternatively, the role of disruption of attachments in the development of depression.

THE NATURE OF IPT

Depression is viewed as having three component processes:

1. *Symptom formation*, which involves the development of depressive affect and the vegetative signs and symptoms, and may derive from psychobiological and/or psychodynamic mechanisms.

2. *Social and interpersonal relations*, which involve interactions in social roles with other persons and which derive from learning based on childhood experiences, concurrent social reinforcement, and/or personal mastery and competence.

3. *Personality*, which involves the enduring traits such as inhibited expression of anger, guilt, poor communication, and/or difficulty with self-esteem. These traits determine the person's unique reactions to interpersonal experience. Personality patterns may provide part of the person's predisposition to episodes of illness and intervenes in the first two processes—symptom formation and social and interpersonal relations. Because of the relatively brief duration of the treatment and the low level of psychotherapeutic intensity, there are few claims that this treatment will have impact upon enduring aspects of personality structure.

IPT facilitates recovery by relieving the depressive symptoms, and by helping the patient develop more productive strategies for dealing with current social and interpersonal problems associated with the onset of symptoms.

The first goal is achieved by educating the patient about the depression; the patient is told that the vague and uncomfortable symptoms of depression are part of a known syndrome that is well-described, well-understood, and relatively common, that it responds to a variety of treatments, and that it has a good prognosis. Psychopharmacologic approaches to alleviate symptoms may be used in conjunction with IPT.

The second goal is achieved by helping the patient understand the interpersonal context of the depression, eg, determining with the patient which of four common problems (grief, role disputes, role transitions, and interpersonal deficits) associated with the onset of depression is related to the patient's depression, and by focusing the psychotherapy around the patient's coping more effectively with the particular problem.

In achieving these goals, reliance is upon techniques such as reassurance, clarification of internal emotional states, improvement of interpersonal communication, and reality testing of perceptions and performance. These techniques conventionally are grouped under the rubric of "supportive" psychotherapy. However, in our view, the term "supportive" psychotherapy is a misnomer. In our view, most of what is called "supportive" psychotherapy attempts to assist the patient to modify his/her interpersonal relations, to change perceptions and cognitions, and to reward specific behaviors.

The main efforts during IPT is on *current* issues at the conscious and preconscious levels. The emphasis is upon current problems, conflicts, frustrations, anxieties, and wishes defined in an interpersonal context. The influence of early childhood experiences is recognized as significant to the presenting problems, but this component is not emphasized in therapy. Rather, an effort is made to define problems in "here-and-now" terms. IPT differs from other psychotherapies in that it is time-limited, focused primarily on the patient's current symptoms of depression and on the interpersonal context associated with the depression. It includes a systematic analysis of relations with "significant others" in the patient's current situation. It has been developed for the treatment of a single disorder—depression. IPT is an *acknowledged* amalgam of many therapeutic techniques. The brevity of the therapy (usually 12 to 16 sessions) precludes major reconstruction of personality, and no assumptions are made about unique personality styles among persons who become depressed.

THE CONDUCT OF IPT

The following material gives a brief outline of IPT:

Goals

1. Reduction of depressive symptoms with restoration of morale and improved self-esteem;
2. Improvement in the quality of the patient's interpersonal relationships and social adjustment by helping him/her develop more effective strategies for dealing with current interpersonal problems.

Methods of Dealing with the Depressive Symptoms

1. Review symptoms and make a diagnosis.
2. Give symptoms a name.
3. Describe depression, its epidemiology, course, prognosis, and treatment.
4. Evaluate the need for medication.
5. Give the patient the "sick role" temporarily.
6. Determine the interpersonal problem areas to be worked on in psychotherapy.

Interpersonal Problems Commonly Associated with Acute Depression

1. *Abnormal Grief Reaction*: refers to depression (not normal bereavement) associated with the death of a significant other. The goals of treatment are to facilitate the delayed mourning process, and to help the patient reestablish interests and relationships that can substitute for that which has been lost.
2. *Interpersonal Role Disputes*: refers to a situation in which the patient and at least one significant other have nonreciprocal expectations about their relationships. The goals of treatment are to help the patient identify the issue(s) in the dispute, to guide the patient in making choices about a plan of action, and to encourage the patient to modify maladaptive communication patterns and/or to reassess expectations in order to bring about a satisfactory resolution to the interpersonal disputes.

3. *Role Transitions*: refers to depression associated with a patient's unsuccessful attempt to cope with life changes. The goals of treatment are to enable the patient to regard the new role(s) in a more positive, less restricted manner, perhaps as an opportunity for growth; and to restore self-esteem by developing in the patient a sense of mastery vis-a-vis demands of the new role.

4. *Interpersonal Deficits*: depression associated with a history of social impoverishment including inadequate or unsustaining interpersonal relationships and poor social skills. Depressed patients who present with a history of severe social isolation tend to be more severely disturbed than those with other presenting problems. The goals are to help the patient identify any past positive relationships and experiences to use a model, to find new situations and persons in which to develop more satisfactory relationships.

EFFICACY DATA ON IPT FOR DEPRESSION

Two controlled clinical trials of IPT for depression, one for acute and one for maintenance outpatient treatment, have been completed and four are underway.

Diagnosis

IPT has been designed for ambulatory patients who meet the criteria of major depression as currently defined by DSM-III or Research Diagnostic Criteria (RDC).

Current efficacy data on IPT in depressed patients are for ambulatory, nonpsychotic, and nonbipolar patients of either sex, and of various racial groups and educational levels. While the earlier trial of IPT was conducted before the availability of RDC or DSM-III diagnostic criteria, on rediagnosis the patients included would meet these criteria. Mentally retarded and chronic alcoholic patients have been excluded from these studies. Persons with personality disorders as defined by the DSM-III or the RDC have not been excluded from efficacy studies.

There has been one trial in opiate addicts in which IPT was added to standard drug abuse program versus drug abuse program alone [30]. The results indicated that IPT did not offer any advantage over standard program in opiate-addicted populations. Thus, the value of IPT or the required modification (if any) with certain personality disorders or other diagnoses requires testing.

IPT as Acute Treatment

The study of the acute treatment of ambulatory depressed men and women compared using IPT alone, amitriptyline alone, and the two in combination against a nonscheduled treatment group for 16 weeks [4]. IPT was administered weekly by experienced psychiatrists. A total of 81 depressed patients entered the randomized treatment study [3,4].

The control for IPT was nonscheduled treatment. In nonscheduled treatment, patients were assigned a psychiatrist whom they were told to contact whenever they felt a need for treatment. No active treatment was scheduled, but the patient could telephone. If his or her needs were of sufficient intensity, a 50-minute session (maximum of one per month) was scheduled. Patients requiring further treatment—and who were still symptomatic after eight weeks, or whose clinical condition had worsened sufficiently to require other treatment—were considered to be failures of this treatment and were withdrawn from the study. This procedure served as an ethically feasible control for psychotherapy in that it allowed a patient to receive periodic supportive help "on demand." Assessments of the patient's clinical condition were made by a clinician who was blind to the treatment the patient was receiving and who did not participate in the clinical phase of the study (the independent clinical evaluator).

IPT as Compared with Nonscheduled Treatment for Acute Treatment

The probability of symptomatic failure over 16 weeks was significantly lower in IPT than in nonscheduled treatment. These results were upheld by a variety of symptom measures made by the independent clinical evaluator, the patient self-report, and the treating psychiatrist. These effects on the patient's social and interpersonal functioning took six to eight months to fully develop. At the one-year follow-up, patients who had received IPT, with or without tricyclics, were functioning at a less impaired level in social activities, with their spouse, children, and other relatives.

IPT as Compared with Tricyclics for Acute Treatment

Overall, the rate of symptomatic improvement was similar to patients receiving IPT alone as compared with tricyclics alone, and both were better than nonscheduled treatment. However, there was a differential effect of the treatments on symptoms [3]. IPT had its impact on improving mood, work performance, interest, suicidal ideation, and guilt. The effects became statistically apparent after four to eight weeks of treatment and were sustained. Amitriptyline had its impact mainly on vegetative signs and symptoms of depression, namely, sleep and appetite disturbance and somatic complaints. The effect on sleep was early, within the first week of treatment.

IPT in Combination with Tricyclics

Because of the differential effects of IPT and tricyclics on the type of symptoms and because patients have a range of symptoms, patients receiving combination treatment as compared with either treatment alone had greater overall improvement in symptoms, lower attrition, and lower chance of symptomatic failure [4]. Patients receiving combination treatment were less likely to refuse it initially and less likely to drop out before the 16 weeks when the study treatment ended. Combination treatment was both more acceptable and better tolerated [31]. There were no negative interactions between drugs and psychotherapy. The effects were additive [32].

Predictors of Response to Acute Treatment

Patients who had an endogenous, nonsituational depression responded best to combined IPT and drugs and less well to IPT alone, which showed no differences in response than did the nonscheduled treatment. The group of patients who received drug alone did somewhere between IPT alone and the combination treatment. Alternatively, patients who had situational nonendogenous depression did equally well on drug alone, IPT alone or the combination and better than on nonscheduled treatment [10,33].

The patient's personality type as measured by a variety of inventories or by the presence of a depressive personality diagnosis according to RDC did not affect response to any of the short-term treatments [34]. This finding suggested that the presence of a personality disorder in addition to major depression does not preclude the use of drugs or IPT for the acute episode.

Follow-Up after Acute Treatment

Patients were followed up one year after treatment had ended. As noted before, patients who had received IPT either alone or in combination were functioning better in social activities, as parents, in the family, and overall [35].

IPT as Maintenance Treatment

IPT as maintenance treatment was tested in an eight-month trial for 150 women recovering from an acute depressive episode who were treated for six to eight weeks with amitriptyline.

This study tested the efficacy of IPT (administered weekly by experienced psychiatric social workers) as compared with a low-contact control (brief monthly visits for assessments), with either amitriptyline, placebo, or no pill; treatment was by random assignment [1].

Maintenance IPT as Compared with Low Contact

The findings showed that maintenance IPT as compared with low contact significantly enhanced social and interpersonal functioning for patients who did not relapse. The effects of IPT on social functioning took six to eight months to become statistically apparent [2]. Patients receiving IPT as compared with low contact were significantly less socially impaired, particularly in work, in their extended families, and in marriage. Overall improvement in social adjustment was significantly greater in IPT than in low contact.

Maintenance IPT as Compared with Tricyclic

Maintenance IPT as compared with amitriptyline was less efficacious in the prevention of symptomatic relapse. Patients receiving amitriptyline only as compared with IPT alone showed less evidence of depressive symptoms during maintenance treatment [36].

Maintenance IPT in Combination with Tricyclic

Because of the differential impact of IPT and of tricyclics on relapse and on social functioning, overall the combination treatment was the most efficacious. Patients who received the combination drug and IPT had a lower risk of relapse and greater improvement in social functioning. Moreover, as was shown for acute treatment, the effects were additive. There were no interactions between drugs and psychotherapy.

Follow-Up After Maintenance Treatment

One and four years after the end of the eight-month maintenance treatment, all patients were followed up. At one year, 30 percent were completely without symptoms, 60 percent had mild return of symptoms over the year, and 10 percent were chronically depressed [37,38]. While the presence of personality problems did not interfere with the short-term treatment, for the long-term outcome, patients who scored high on the neurotic personality scale and who did not receive maintenance treatment of either drugs or of IPT were doing less well [39].

CLINICAL TRIALS OF IPT IN PROGRESS

There are currently four studies in progress testing out the efficacy of IPT in ambulatory depressed patient [5]. These are:

1. A multi-site NIMH-sponsored collaborative study on the treatment of depression testing the efficacy of IPT, cognitive therapy, imipramine and clinical management, placebo and clinical management for 16 weeks in 240 ambulatory depressed patients at three sites (George Washington University, University of Pittsburgh, University of Oklahoma) [40].

2. A separate study at the University of Pittsburgh testing out the efficacy of maintenance IPT alone, IPT and placebo, IPT and imipramine, clinical management and imipramine, clinical management and placebo in 125 ambulatory patients with recurrent depression administered over a three-year period [5].

3. A study at the University of Southern California testing the efficacy of noritriptyline placebo/IPT in 60 to 90 ambulatory depressed elderly patients over 16 weeks.

4. A study at the University of Wisconsin testing the efficacy of CB group with or without homework, IPT, or waiting list in 140 depressed outpatients for ten weeks.

Because of the enduring nature of marital problems in depressed patient [41,42] and the tendency for patients with marital problems to have enduring symptoms [43], the Yale group is currently developing a manual for IPT in a conjoint marital context. After the development and pilot testing of this manual and the training of therapists we will test out the efficacy of individual versus conjoint marital IPT for depressed patients with marital problems.

CONCLUSION

IPT is a short-term, interpersonal psychotherapy designed specifically for depressed patients, defined in a procedural manual, and tested in two clinical trials. A training program for experienced therapists interested in undertaking research in its use has been developed. IPT has been refined further since the studies were completed and is now being tested outside of the New Haven-Boston Centers where it was developed.

In two clinical trials with ambulatory nonbipolar major depressive patients, we have demonstrated that for acute treatment, IPT as compared with nonscheduled treatment was more efficacious for symptom reduction and later in enhancing social functioning and was about equal to tricyclic therapy in symptom reduction. For maintenance treatment, IPT compared with low contact therapy in recovering patients was more efficacious for enhancing social and interpersonal functioning. IPT was not as good as tricyclics in the prevention of relapse. The effects on social functioning take at least six to eight months to become apparent. In both the acute and the maintenance studies, the combination of IPT and tricyclic therapy was better than either treatment alone. For the endogenous-nonsituational depressive patient, IPT alone did not offer anything above no scheduled treatment. There was some suggestion that IPT had some enduring effect on social functioning one year after treatment ended and that the presence of personality problems did not affect short-term outcome. The results of the four studies currently underway in Centers which did not develop IPT will provide more definitive information on its efficacy.

ACKNOWLEDGMENTS

The development and testing of IPT has been supported over the years by grant numbers MH137838, MH15650, MH26466, and MH26467 from the Psychopharmacology Research Branch, Clinical Research Branch of the National Institute of Mental Health, Alcohol, Drug Abuse and Mental Health Administration, and from grant number MH33827-03 from the Psychosocial Treatments Research Branch, of the National Institute of Mental Health.

This work has involved the efforts of many people over the years, particularly the late Alberto DiMascio, PhD, who led the Boston portion of this project; Brigitte Prusoff, PhD, who was in charge of the data analysis for the two clinics; Carlos Neu, MD, who assisted in the earlier versions of the IPT manual; and Eve Chevron and Bruce Rounsaville, MD, who developed the latest version of the IPT manual and developed and carried out the IPT training program. Irene Waskow, PhD, in her role as director of the NIMH Collaborative Study on the Treatment of Depression, which included IPT as one of the treatments, gave us the impetus to further refine the treatment and develop the training.

Portions of this manuscript appeared in Klerman GL and Weissman MM: Interpersonal Theory and Research. In Rush AJ (ed): *Short-Term Therapies for Depression: Behavioral, Interpersonal, Cognitive and Psychodynamic Approaches.* New York: Guilford Press, 1982, pp. 88-104.

REFERENCES

1. Klerman GL, DiMascio A, Weissman MM, Prusoff BA, Paykel ES: Treatment of depression by drugs and psychotherapy. *Am J Psychiatry* 131:186-191, 1974
2. Weissman MM, Klerman GL, Paykel ES, Prusoff BA, Hanson B: Treatment effects on the social adjustment of depressed patients. *Arch Gen Psychiatry* 30:771-778, 1974
3. DiMascio A, Weissman MM, Prusoff BA, Neu C, Zwilling M, Klerman GL: Differential symptom reduction by drugs and psychotherapy in acute depression. *Arch Gen Psychiatry* 36:1450-1456, 1979
4. Weissman MM, Prusoff BA, DiMascio A, Neu C, Goklaney M, Klerman GL: The efficacy of drugs and psychotherapy in the treatment of acute depressive episodes. *Am J Psychiatry* 136(No.4B):555-558, 1979
5. Weissman MM: The psychological treatment of depression: an update of clinical trials. In *Psychotherapy Research: Where We Are and Where Should We Go?* Edited by Spitzer RL, Williams JBW. New York: Guilford Press, 1984
6. Klerman GL, Rounsaville B, Chevron E, Neu C, Weissman M: *Manual for Short-Term Interpersonal Psychotherapy (IPT) of Depression.* Unpublished manuscript, 1982
7. Meyer A: *Psychobiology: A Science of Man.* Springfield, Charles C Thomas, 1957
8. Sullivan HS: *Conceptions of Modern Psychiatry.* New York: Norton, 1953a
9. Sullivan HS: *The Interpersonal Theory of Psychiatry.* New York: Norton, 1953b
10. Cohen MB, Baker G, Cohen RA, Fromm-Reichmann F, Weigert EA: An intensive study of twelve cases of manic-depressive psychoses. *Psychiatry* 17:103-137, 1954
11. Arieti S, Bemporad J: *Severe and Mild Depression: The Psychotherapeutic Approach.* New York: Basic Books, 1978
12. Becker J: *Depression: Theory and Research.* New York: Wiley, 1974

164   M. M. Weissman and G. L. Klerman

13. Chodoff P: The core problem in depression. In *Science and Psychoanalysis*, edited by Masserman J. New York: Grune and Stratton, 1970
14. Frank JD: Psychotherapy: the restoration of morale. *Am J Psychiatry* 131:271-274, 1974
15. Bowlby J: *Attachment and Loss*. London: Hogarth, 1969
16. Bowlby J: The making and breaking of affectional bonds: II. Some principles of psychotherapy. *Br J Psychiatry* 130:421-431, 1977
17. Rutter M: *Maternal Deprivation Reassessed*. London: Penguin, 1972
18. Henderson S, Byrne DG, Duncan-Jones P, et al: Social bonds in the epidemiology of neurosis. *Br J Psychiatry* 132:463-466, 1978
19. Brown GW, Harris T, Copeland JR: Depression and loss. *Br J Psychiatry* 130:1-18, 1977
20. Miller P, Ingham JG: Friends, confidants and symptoms. *Soc Psychiatry* 11:51-58, 1976
21. Holmes TH, Goodell H, Wolf S: *The Nose: An Experimental Study of Reactions within the Nose in Human Subjects During Varying Life Experiences*. Springfield, Il: Charles C Thomas, 1950
22. Paykel ES, Myers JK, Dienelt MN, et al: Life events and depression: a controlled study. *Arch Gen Psychiatry* 21:753-760, 1969
23. Ilfeld FW: Current social stressors and symptoms of depression. *Am J Psychiatry* 134:161-166, 1977
24. Pearlin LI, Lieberman MA: Social sources of emotional distress. In *Research In Community and Mental Health*, edited by Simmons R. Greenwich CT: JAI, 1979
25. Bloom BL, Asher SJ, White SW: Marital disruption as a stressor: a review and analysis. *Psychol Bull* 85:867-894, 1978
26. Weissman MM, Paykel ES: *The Depressed Woman: A Study of Social Relationships*. Chicago: University of Chicago Press, 1974
27. Briscoe CW, Smith JB: Depression and marital turmoil. *Arch Gen Psychiatry* 28:811-817, 1973
28. Kreitman N, Collins J, Nelson B, et al: Neurosis and marital interaction: I. Personality and symptoms. *Br J Psychiatry* 117:33-46, 1970
29. Coyne JC: Depression and the response of others. *J Abnor Psychology* 85:186-193, 1976
30. Rounsaville BJ, Glazer W, Weissman MM, Wilber CH, Kleber HD: Short-term interpersonal psychotherapy in methadone maintained opiate addicts. *Arch Gen Psychiatry*, in press.
31. Herceg-Baron RL, Prusoff BA, Weissman MM, DiMascio A, Neu C, Klerman GL: Pharmacotherapy and psychotherapy in acutely depressed patients: a study of attrition patterns in a clinical trial. *Compr Psychiatry* 20(4):315-325, 1979
32. Rounsaville BJ, Weissman MM, Klerman GL: Do psychotherapy and pharmacotherapy for depression conflict? Empirical evidence from a clinical trial. *Arch Gen Psychiatry* 38:24-29, 1981
33. Prusoff BA, Weissman MM, Klerman GL, Rounsaville BJ: Research diagnostic criteria of depression: Their role as predictors of differential response to psychotherapy and drug treatment. *Arch Gen Psychiatry* 37:796-803, 1980
34. Zuckerman DM, Prusoff BA, Weissman MM, Padian NS: Personality as a predictor of psychotherapy and pharmacotherapy outcome for depressed outpatients. *J Consult Clin Psychol* 48(6):730-735, 1980

35. Weissman MM, Klerman GL, Prusoff BA, Sholomskas D, Padian N: Depressed outpatients: results one year after treatment with drugs and/or interpersonal psychotherapy. *Arch Gen Psychiatry* 38:51-55, 1981
36. Paykel ES, DiMascio A, Klerman GL, Prusoff BA, and Weissman MM: Maintenance therapy of depression. *Pharmakopsychiatrie Neuro-Psychopharmakologie* 9:127-136, 1976
37. Weissman MM, Kasl SV, Klerman GL: Follow-up of depressed women after maintenance treatment. *Am J Psychiatry*, 133(7):757-760, 1976
38. Weissman MM, Klerman GL: The chronic depressive in the community: Unrecognized and poorly treated. *Compr Psychiatry* 18(6):523-532, 1977
39. Weissman MM, Prusoff BA, Klerman GL: Personality and the prediction of long-term outcome of depression. *Am J Psychiatry* 135(7):797-800, 1978
40. NIMH Treatment of Depression Collaborative Research (Pilot Phase). Revised Research Plan, Psychosocial Treatments Research Branch, NIMH Rockville, Maryland, January 1980
41. Rounsaville BJ, Weissman MM, Prusoff BA, Herceg-Baron RL: Marital disputes and treatment outcome in depressed women. *Compr Psychiatry* 20:483-490, 1979
42. Rounsaville BJ, Weissman MM, Prusoff BA, Herceg-Baron R: Process of psychotherapy among depressed women with marital disputes. *Am J Orthopsychiatry* 49(3):505-510, 1979
43. Rounsaville BJ, Prusoff BA, Weissman MM: The course of marital disputes in depressed women: a 48-month follow-up study. *Compr Psychiatry* 21(2):111--118, 1980

CHAPTER 9

Schizophrenia: The Interaction of Family and Neuroleptic Therapy

Michael J. Goldstein

THE IMPACT OF BRIEF HOSPITALIZATION ON THE AFTERCARE AND TREATMENT OF SCHIZOPHRENIA

The last 15 years have witnessed a marked diminution in the length of inpatient hospitalization for schizophrenic patients. While hospitalization was previously measured in units of months or even years, current practice involves an average of two to three weeks for an acute episode of a schizophrenic disorder. In some extreme examples, as in overburdened county hospitals, patients are released after a matter of a few days of inpatient care. The period of inpatient treatment for schizophrenia is governed more by economic than therapeutic considerations, such as the limits of coverage from third party payers, or by governmental units. This truncation of in-patient stay has received support from studies such as that by Glick and associates [1], which found few, if any, benefits for most schizophrenics beyond the five-week average used with their short-term hospitalization group. Ironically, since the time that study was completed, their short-term hospitalization condition would now define a long-term condition in any contemporary clinical research project. Empirical evidence concerning the impact of still briefer hospitalization periods is largely lacking.

The variability in hospitalization periods is an important consideration in evaluating the role and impact of any facet of a comprehensive aftercare program. Depending on the length of stay and aggressiveness of the inpatient treatment program, patients are discharged in highly variable states of partial remission. Thus, for some patients the aftercare pharmacotherapy involves the continuous administration of the standard dose used during the inpatient period, while for patients who have been hospitalized for longer periods and achieved a reasonable degree of remission, the strategy for aftercare might involve a tapering down of the phenothiazine dose level to what is termed a maintenance dose level. Because hospital stays are so brief in some settings, many writers have suggested that the treatment of schizophrenia be considered as a three-phase process—inpatient acute treatment, outpatient stabilization, and aftercare maintenance. The problem with this distinction is defining the stabilization phase with clear clinical criteria. For example, in two recent studies [2,3], stabilization was believed to have been achieved by four to six weeks after discharge in the former, but by six months postdischarge in the latter. Thus, one person's total treatment period may merely be another's stabilization period.

This difficulty in defining stabilization poses serious problems for the design and interpretation of studies trying to evaluate the impact of variations in antipsychotic dose levels during the after-care period. The question of whether maintenance dose levels of phenothiazine drugs can be substantially lower than current practice suggests, or might be permissible when combined with an effective psychosocial program, will be answered very differently depending upon when such a program is initiated. In one study [4], the transition from a standard dose to a very low dose of injectable fluphena-zine (1.5 to 5 mg) took place after one year of posthospitalization treatment. One year posthospitalization is hardly the optimal time for the introduction of a psychosocial intervention program in a study designed to test for interactions between phenothiazine dose level and the impact of such a program. Neither is it an optimal period to provide support for a family which has been coping with the reentry of a mentally ill relative for that year. Even if such a study reported positive results of the combined pharmaco-and psychosocial therapy, it would not bear on the issue of whether a similar lower dose level combined with an effective psychosocial program would be appropriate for the immediate posthospitalization period. This may seem like a very obvious point, yet it frequently clouds the interpretation of studies dealing with the impact of uni-modal and multimodal aftercare treatments.

The release of schizophrenic patients into the community after relatively brief inpatient stays, frequently requires that family members reabsorb the patients back into their homes and take on a primary caretaker's role. Mostly, family members are ill prepared for such a role and receive little guidance from mental health professionals as to appropriate roles and behaviors. Since research originally carried out in Great Britain [5,6] indicates that the emotional climate of the family influences the likelihood that a patient can survive without relapse for at least nine months after hospital discharge, there is considerable interest in developing family-based intervention programs to foster a therapeutic home environment. Such programs typically are initiated while the patient is hospitalized or shortly thereafter, and continue through the aftercare period. The initial positive reports of such programs [7–9] have not only raised the optimism of clinicians regarding psychosocial interventions for schizophrenics and their families, but have raised the question of whether the traditional mode of maintenance pharmacotherapy can be substantially modified in terms of dose level, patterning, or duration when combined with an efficacious family intervention program. Little empirical evidence exists on this issue of potential drug-family therapy interactions, and clinical research on this topic is sorely needed.

MAINTENANCE DRUG THERAPY: ALTERNATIVE MODELS

There is little question that a regular program of maintenance pharmacotherapy carried out from nine months to one year after hospital discharge greatly forestalls relapse. The study by Hogarty et al [3], which insured compliance through the use of fluphenazine deconoate, found a relapse rate of 68 percent in placebo-treated patients and 38 percent in drug-treated patients over a one-year period. Similar results, with an even sharper differential between drug and placebo condition, was found by Kane et al [10] in a sample of first admission cases. Across a number of studies [7,10,11], it appears that young schizophrenic patients rated as having a poor premorbid history (limited social and heterosexual relationships) are particularly prone to relapse without maintenance pharmacotherapy. The drug response pattern of patients with a good premorbid history is not so clear. In the Goldstein et al study, in which patients were randomly assigned to moderate (25 mg) or low doses (6.25 mg) of fluphenazine enanthate, patients with a poor premorbid history relapsed readily on the lower dose, while good premorbids had a low rate of relapse on both, and showed less depressive symptomatology when on the lower dose. In the Marder et al study, patients were assigned to a clinically appropriate dose level after a 30-day wash-out period from prior phenothiazine treatment. Good premorbid patients were more likely to show improvement during the drug withdrawal period and to require a significantly lower maintenance drug dose level after discharge than did poor premorbid patients.

While the results are quite clear concerning the value of maintenance pharmacotherapy, particularly for schizophrenic patients with a poor premorbid history, there are a number of disquieting and unresolved issues regarding this aspect of aftercare treatment. First, while maintenance pharmacotherapy reduces, in stock market terms, the "downside" risk of relapse, it does not foster effective social recovery. In fact, there are suggestions in the literature that the continued presence of so-called negative symptoms, postpsychotic depression, or what Huber [12] terms the "reine defect," may be conditioned or prolonged by continued drug treatment. Further, the very real risk of tardive dyskinesia, which is heightened by continuous drug treatment, has led clinicians and researchers to desire alternative pharmacologic treatment strategies that can still protect against relapse, while minimizing the social risk of this type of amotivational syndrome and the physical risk of tardive dyskinesia. Two general strategies have been suggested, one characterized by the intermittent use of medication, and a second by the utilization of substantially lower doses than those conventionally used, which are supplemented by some form of psychosocial intervention.

The former strategy, associated with the work of Carpenter and his colleagues [13], builds on the work of Manfred Bleuler, in which patients are placed on a drug-free regimen after remission (and stabilization) from an index episode; however, patients are placed on an aggressive pharmacotherapy regimen when incipient signs of the illness appear. This drug therapy is continued until the episode appears to have been aborted and then the patient is weaned once again to a drug-free state. Carpenter uses the term *targeted medication* to describe such a program. In this program, patients referred to their aftercare clinic, after hospitalization, are placed on a drug-withdrawal program for a 30-day period. Evidence to date suggests that 70 percent of the patients, who are drawn from a very chronic pool of cases, will survive this "wash-out" period. Those patients who do not survive this period are placed on medication and rotated again to a drug-free regimen after they have stabilized. Those patients who survive such a withdrawal period are kept on a drug-free program for as long as possible, a program amply enriched by individual, group, family, and occupational therapy [14]. Drug therapy is reinstated at the first sign of the return of psychotic symptoms. A key element in such a program is the determination of the incipient signs of psychosis for each patient. Both patients and key relatives are trained in the recognition of these incipient signs and symptoms and are encouraged to reinstitute drug therapy as soon as they appear. Heinrichs and Carpenter [14] report that cooperation with such a program is, in fact, enhanced when the patient has experienced a recrudescence of symptoms while under the care of their aftercare treatment program. Both patients and relatives are then unable to deny that relapse is a possibility and are sensitized to the incipient signs of an episode. The research by Herz and Melville [15] who also advocate a program of intermittent drug therapy, have identified a clustering of incipient nonpsychotic signs of a schizophrenic episode, which can be utilized by clinicians, patients, and relatives to recognize signs and symptoms of probable relapse.

It is unclear, at this time, how many patients can be maintained on an intermittent program or whether, when incipient signs appear, patients on the verge of psychosis are readily induced to begin drug therapy once again. However, preliminary results are encouraging.

The second alternative involves the use of continuous pharmacotherapy, but at substantially lower dose levels than was common in previous clinical practice. As indicated in the beginning of this chapter, there is considerable variation as to when dose reductions are likely to occur: immediately after discharge, after stabilization, or after a year of maintenance drug therapy. In one study [7], patients were randomly assigned to two dose levels: 6.25 and 25 mg of injectable fluphenazine enanthate begun immediately after discharge from a community mental health center after an average of 12 days of inpatient care. The controlled trial lasted for six weeks, after which clinicians were free to prescribe the drug or dose of their choice. The relapse rate was 24 percent for the lower dose, no family therapy condition and 10 percent for the comparable higher dose group. Despite the wide variability in treatment after the controlled period, these differences persisted and were enhanced at the time of a six-month follow-up (48 versus 17 percent). Thus, it appears that a 6.25 mg dose is below the threshold of relapse protection for the average patient who has been hospitalized for a relatively brief period, and who has not been through a posthospitalization stabilization regimen. While not appropriate for all patients, it should be noted that for some with a good premorbid history, this dose is a reasonable starting point.

In one study by Hogarty [3], the median dose of fluphenazine decanoate after stabilization was 12.5 mg every 14 days. In an ongoing study by Nuechterlein [16], this same dose was used after an average four-week tapering down period in a fixed dose design, and data so far indicate that two thirds of the patients in the study survived the one-year follow-up period without relapsing. Thus, this drug dosage represents a reasonable starting point for the aftercare utilization of fluphenazine deconoate. While the low dose used in the Goldstein et al study seems below the threshold for successful maintenance of a recently discharged schizophrenic patient hospitalized for a very brief period, we cannot assume that such a low dose is ineffective after an extended period of stabilization on a higher dose. In a previously cited study [4], Kane et al transferred half of the sample of patients who had been stabilized in the community for an average of 64 weeks into the community on a dose range of 12.5 to 50 mg of fluphenazine deconoate to a low-dose regimen of the same drug involving a one-tenth dose reduction (1.25 to 5 mg). This is a very considerable reduction in dose level. These investigators reported that patients treated with this very low dose of neuroleptic drug are likely to relapse during a one-year treatment period. Twenty-six of 62 patients assigned to the low-dose condition relapsed, although only seven required rehospitalization. Among the 64 patients continued on the standard dose, three patients relapsed a total of four times. However, relapse is not the only issue. More patients, continued on the standard dose, showed signs of presumptive tardive dyskinesia or ratings of abnormal movements on the Simpson Dyskinesia Scale.

All patients who showed signs of relapse were treated with a standard dose and then returned to their assigned dose thereafter.

Those low-dose patients who were put back into the study and completed the one-year follow-up received significantly less total phenothiazine medication than did the patients taking the standard dose.

Interestingly, ratings of social adjustment and family burden revealed, that despite the increased risk of relapse, the low-dose patients were not significantly worse off than the standard-dose patients and were in fact doing *better* in some areas.

The next step in this type of research is to determine whether a family intervention program can permit schizophrenic patients to survive in the community on such a low dose. Therefore, the next section of this chapter reviews some attributes of current family intervention programs.

FAMILY INTERVENTION PROGRAMS

Brief Crisis-Oriented Family Therapy

Crisis-oriented family therapy was designed to support acute schizophrenics and their families during the difficult period of social reimmersion. Typically leaving the hospital in a state of partial remission, patients are especially vulnerable to the inevitable tensions of returning to a family recently disrupted by a psychotic breakdown. Other family members are also under considerable duress and may find it hard to support the patient. First, they have had to cope with the decompensation of a relative and often suffer guilt over provoking it; now, they must bear the responsibility of caring for a residually symptomatic schizophrenic. The potential for conflict is high, as is the patient's vulnerability to it.

Crisis-oriented family therapy attempts to manage the potentially disruptive events of this period effectively and to minimize stress for the patient. During the high-risk postdischarge period, the patient and family members meet with a therapist, in six weekly sessions, for shared problem solving. The sessions primarily concentrate on current circumstances that participants identify as particularly stressful to the patient. Treatment is directed toward identifying problematic situations, avoiding them when possible, and assuaging the destructive impact of them when they occur. Thus, the therapy is brief, concrete, and problem-focused.

Preliminary Topics in Treatment

Although the topics addressed in therapy vary considerably, dictated by the particular needs of each family, two foci are initially appropriate in the majority of cases. The first is that of unrealistic expectations about the length of recovery. Usually, expectations are overly positive. The patient or relatives may believe that work and school should be resumed almost immediately. Such expectations translate into demands exceeding the patient's functional capacity, jeopardizing stability, and leading the patient and relatives to anger and hopelessness when failure is encountered. Occasionally, there is unwarranted pessimism about the patient's long-term prospects, leading to despair and resignation. In both cases, the therapist must help in setting modest short-term expectations while bolstering hope for the long term.

Patients and relatives are informed from the start that full recovery often takes six months to a year, and that premature pressure on patients can be gravely counterproductive. Frequently, this theme requires reiteration over the course of treatment. To minimize discouragement, the therapist can highlight progress from week to week, however slight it may be. The concept of the "internal yardstick" suggested by Anderson, Meisel, and Houpt [17] can be helpful in sensitizing patients and families to small increments of progress.

The need to correct unrealistic expectations is illustrated in the case of Mark. This patient's parents found it very difficult to accept the fact that Mark slept for much of the day and, when awake, stayed close to home. The therapist had to remind the parents and the patient repeatedly that this was normal and necessary for a fragile and medicated schizophrenic patient in the early phases of recovery.

Mrs. S.: Mark still sleeps the whole day. He never goes out and he's always tired.
Therapist: Well, very often after hospitalization like this, people tend to sleep an awful lot. It's important for them to be calm and quiet and take good care of themselves. So his sleeping is a good sign. How do you feel about it, Mark?
Mark: I'm just not ready to go out. I get too nervous.
Therapist: You feel you need more time to just relax.
Mrs. S.: But I think it's important for him to see people again.
Mark: Well, I went to day treatment this week. I saw people again.

Therapist: So you went to day treatment. That's really a positive step! Last week you didn't want to go anywhere.

A second topic in therapy is each participant's experience of the events leading up to and during the schizophrenic decompensation. I have found that therapists rarely inquire about the subjective reactions of patients and their families to these events. Hence, important feelings are neglected, while the breakdown is often perceived as shameful. Discussion of the schizophrenic episode desensitizes family members to the behavioral manifestations of florid psychosis, allowing them to acknowledge odd behavior exhibited by the patient. Open conversation also permits the treatment participants to validate their perceptions of specific symptomatology, helping them recognize the signs of an incipient breakdown should future regressions occur. Of primary importance, though, are the feelings of empathy and relief for both patients and relatives that grow from sharing what had been confusing, frightening, and commonly alienating experiences. These points are illustrated by the case of Steve, who described an intensely emotional experience that he had previously been too ashamed and confused to discuss.

Steve: I was waiting in the airport to go to Vietnam and I couldn't stand it. I started shaking and I couldn't breathe and I couldn't think.
Therapist: That sounds so frightening. You must have been in a panic. That happens some times when people are really afraid.
Steve: Yeah, um . . . (crying) . . . Well, I saw this Oriental girl and I . . . um . . . couldn't stop thinking about her and I went to the bathroom and I wouldn't come out. I started to masturbate and just kept getting more and more frightened. They (the military police) came to get me and I wouldn't leave (still crying). This is so hard for me to say. I don't want to talk about it any more.
Therapist: I know it must be so hard. But there are times when it's important for you to talk about it. When terrifying things happen, sometimes we do things that we wouldn't ordinarily do. Going to Vietnam is a very frightening thing.
Mother: It's alright, Steve. You have to let it out.
Steve: I didn't want to tell you.
Mother: It's okay. I'm glad you told me. I never knew what you went through (crying).

As this dialogue shows, discussion can help the family appreciate the full impact of stress on the patient and often fosters a more empathetic, supportive set.

Exploration of the psychotic break also serves to prepare the family for the remainder of treatment. Relatives often gain awareness of how severe the patient's disturbance really is, an awareness that can be utilized in setting more realistic expectations regarding the course of recovery. Beyond recognizing that the patient really does need help, family members often realize the importance of their role in assisting the patient.

Perhaps most significantly, exploration of the psychosis usually reveals connections between stressful events and decompensation. Directing attention to stressors that precipitated the breakdown, the therapist explains that stress may trigger psychotic episodes. Parenthetically, when a family member is part of a precipitating event, it is imperative that the event and not the relative be labeled the stressor, thus avoiding unnecessary blame and guilt. In discussing the potential for stress to exacerbate schizophrenia, the value of preventing and adequately coping with stressful life events is introduced. Finally, the therapist briefly explains the treatment rationale of improving coping skills to promote recovery and avert regressions.

Four Sequential Therapeutic Objectives

After the preliminary work of (1) suggesting realistic recovery expectations, (2) exploring the psychosis, and (3) explicating the rationale for stress-management, crisis-oriented family therapy is oriented toward the attainment of four objectives. Briefly, the objectives involve (1) identifying the two or three current, most hazardous stressors threatening the patient, (2) developing strategies to prevent stress and cope with these, (3) having families implement the strategies, and refine them, and, (4) engaging in anticipatory planning to prevent and cope with future stresses. These objectives are pursued sequentially, with the latter activities dependent on those previously accomplished.

Objective 1: Identifying Stressors The initial objective of identifying situations stressful to the patient is pursued in three steps. First, each participant is asked to list current circumstances that subject the patient to stress. Second, these stressors are briefly discussed, leading to agreement on the two or three most threatening to the patient's stability. Finally, the most threatening stressors are explored in detail, yielding specific and concrete descriptions of each stressor. These two or three stressors subsequently become the focus of therapy.

The identification of stressors often begins with considering whether problems that precipitated the schizophrenic episode are still creating difficulty. Precipitating stressors are first explored because of their apparent capacity for disruption. They may also serve as vivid examples of the kind of situations therapy participants are expected to identify. After determining whether precipitating factors remain problematic, each participant is encouraged to identify other situations that threaten the patient now or in the immediate future. Patients and their relatives commonly respond by mentioning broad and general problems. Pervasive patient-relative conflict, job or school concerns, drug abuse, and religious cult involvement exemplify the sorts of stressors frequently noted.

Frequently, patients and relatives are quick to criticize and blame one another during these discussions. This activity can be exceedingly destructive and must be avoided. Often, family members need assistance in learning to express requests and opinions without criticism and blaming. Training in communication skills can assist the family members in making requests of one another without provoking conflict. A discussion of interpersonal tension is often an appropriate time to develop these skills. Finally, the therapist should conclude the exploration of each stressor by checking to ensure that the final account is understood and acceptable to all involved.

Objective 2: Developing Stress Prevention and Coping Strategies
Devising plans to prevent and cope with disruptive life events is the second objective in treatment. Prevention strategies are designed to avoid the patient's exposure to stressful situations or to minimize the destructive impact when prevention fails.

Prevention strategies are intended to protect the patient from hazards by encouraging him to avoid exposure to noxious events. These plans may prescribe action for the patient, relatives, or both. Some prevention plans have the patient prepare for or avoid specific activities (eg, the patient is instructed to find out about a movie before attending it to avoid terrifying or bloody scenes). Similarly, prevention plans may mandate certain action from a relative (as when a family member is to cease asking the patient about returning to work) or from more than one family member (as when parents are asked to avoid arguments in the patient's presence).

Prevention strategies often address conflict between the patient and a family member. Plans may call for reducing contact between conflict-prone parties; others restrict specific sorts of contact, including particular conversations or interaction in certain problematic situations (eg, when the father is rushing off to work). Still others focus on defusing interpersonal tension as it begins and preventing escalation into destructive interchanges.

Residual schizophrenic symptoms and family reactions to them comprise a common source of conflict. Hallucinations, delusions, social withdrawal, excessive sleeping, and other symptoms are typical at this point in recovery. Relatives often react critically to the symptoms, and such reactions frequently lead to more generalized interpersonal tension. Since symptoms are largely beyond the patient's control, prevention strategies concentrate on the interpersonal consequences rather than on the symptoms.

Coping plans become important when strategies for prevention fail and the patient encounters stress-producing circumstances. Sometimes, coping plans involve the relatives. They may be called upon to terminate stressful interactions, to engage a mediator to resolve a dispute peacefully, to intervene in arguments between the patient and another, or to offer the patient emotional support in the aftermath of a disturbing experience. However, coping plans that can be utilized by the patient are especially emphasized, for they provide the schizophrenic patient with badly needed means of self-protection.

Objective 3: Implementing and Evaluating Stress Control Strategies Implementing, evaluating, and improving the stress prevention and coping strategies is the third therapy objective. Participants are instructed to implement the strategies as soon as circumstances permit. Shortcomings of the plans are frequently revealed as the family attempts to follow them. Failure to implement the strategies may also be found. In this phase of treatment, obstacles to successful stress prevention and coping are identified and overcome.

When patients and relatives employ the new strategies, they often encounter difficulties. To assure continued effort, therapists may reinforce the attempts with praise and underscore any benefits that were reaped. The next step is obtaining a description of the attempt so the strategies can be made more effective. Sometimes a minor adjustment or elaboration is all a plan requires. Other times, strategies may need substantial modification or even replacement. The nature and extent of alternation depends on how successful the original strategy was and what would be necessary to correct its insufficiencies. The process of refining a strategy is basically the same as creating one (see Objective 2), with the exception that development revolves around aspects of the strategy that require modification.

Sound stress prevention or coping strategies can fail if the person carrying them out lacks requisite psychosocial skills. Problems of skill deficits are most likely with the patient, a schizophrenic in the early stages of restitution. When plans require an awareness of one's impact on others, assertiveness, or the recognition of emotions (to name but a few) the patient may find them unmanageable. Significant others may also be unable to implement strategies, especially when the plans call for inhibiting criticism and anger or for empathizing with the patient. Rarely will treatment participants recognize what is awry in these situations, so the therapist must be particularly alert for skill limitations. When crucial skills are absent, a strategy that does not demand them may be developed. Alternatively, necessary skills can sometimes be developed through instruction, modeling, coaching, and practice within the treatment sessions. Whether to switch to a less demanding strategy or to develop specific skills depends on the relative expediency of the two possibilities, their relative chances for success, and secondary benefits that may result from skill acquisition.

Failure to implement a stress prevention or coping plan is another common problem. This may occur for a number of reasons, and determining the basis for noncompliance is usually the first step in eliminating it. Individuals who fail to enact a strategy may not understand what is expected of them, in which case a careful explanation is in order. They may find some aspect of the strategy unacceptable; either their objection must be worked through by discussion, or the plan must be altered. Sometimes, cues for enactment are not recognized, and a detailed examination of when to implement the strategy is required. Finally, motivation for utilizing the plan may be insufficient. This calls for reducing the "costs" of implementation by amending the plan and/or reemphasizing the importance of protecting the patient from stress. It should be remembered that family members often feel badly about these failures, so therapists must handle implementation problems with tact and sensitivity.

Objective 4: Anticipatory Planning The fourth treatment objective, anticipatory planning, prepares the patient for taxing events likely to transpire in the months after therapy. Anticipatory planning includes identifying potentially disruptive upcoming events and devising prevention and coping strategies for managing them. This final stage in treatment consists of repeating the first two objectives, only this time with future stressors rather than current ones.

As patients recover, they may resume employment, education, dating, or other social contacts; grow progressively independent, perhaps move to their own apartment; and generally assume increasing responsibilities. Sometimes they regress and suffer acute symptoms, and may even be rehospitalized. Anticipatory planning is conducted to help prepare the patient for the challenges ahead by recognizing potential problems and devising plans to control them. The actual format of this preparatory work is essentially the same as for the first two objectives. First, stressors are identified and analyzed into stress events. Second, stress prevention and coping strategies are devised.

Longer-Term Family Intervention

Subsequent family programs which have appeared in the literature have been more extensive than those developed by Goldstein et al. This seems at least partially due to the fact that they have been developed for a more chronic schizophrenic patient who may, in fact, have had a number of prior episodes. It remains to be seen whether families of patients undergoing their first lifetime episode of schizophrenia are readily engaged in such a long-term commitment. The extended family intervention programs do differ notably in certain formal properties, varying from those in which the relatives are the primary target of the intervention [9], to those where the patient is continuously present from family education onward [8]. Most programs do last a minimum of nine months postdischarge and have provisions for a maintenance phase lasting up to two years. Thus, these programs, which involve continuous maintenance medication, represent a major commitment of the institution to the family and vice versa. It is not clear from published reports how many families refuse to make such long-term commitments. However, a number of writers [8,18] indicate that few families withdraw from such a program after the early sessions. The details of these extended programs are described by Goldstein [19].

Regardless of the orientation of the program initiators, all extended family programs operate from the premise that there is a strong relationship between patient vulnerability and family anxiety or behaviors. Thus, these programs are designed to accomplish two goals: decrease the patient's vulnerability to stimuli through a program of maintenance chemotherapy, and decrease the intensity of the family environment through a program of support, information, structure, and specific coping mechanisms for dealing with a partially remitted psychotic family member. Most programs involve family sessions which are structured to some degree and involve a directive therapeutic attitude designed to increase the predictability and stability of the family environment.

The therapeutic models guiding these activities vary from the behavioral approach of Falloon et al [2], which combines communication and problem-solving training in social skills carried out in a family context, to the Anderson, Hogarty and Reiss [20] model, which draws loosely from structural family therapy concepts to emphasize the importance of encouraging boundary and intergenerational differentiation. Despite these quite different orientations, most extended intervention programs emphasize highly structured, low-key family sessions initiated as soon as the acute phase of the illness has been controlled. Most therapies reinforce family boundaries and encourage the gradual (but not premature) resumption of responsibility by the patient. Both the Anderson and Falloon programs involve the use of some form of "homework" through which family members are encouraged to support the gradual assumption of social role functioning by the patient. Despite notable differences in specific theoretical orientation, both the Falloon and Anderson approaches operate broadly within what has been termed the family systems model, as they emphasize the need for reciprocal changes in behavior by all family members participating in the program.

One thing that characterizes all extended family programs for schizophrenia is the critical importance of therapist control of the affective intensity in the sessions. The expression of affect, particularly negative affect of the high expressed emotion (EE) type [21], which may be valued in some therapeutic contexts, is actively discouraged and/or interrupted by the therapist. The vulnerability of schizophrenic patients to affective and critical messages, demands this stance. In addition, such incidents provide the therapist with an opportunity to model more appropriate ways of handling intrafamilial conflict.

Impact of Family Education Programs

Controlled trials involving family intervention programs have revealed very impressive results in terms of relapse reduction. Figure 1 represents the relapse rates from the three controlled trials, published as of this writing, one with a six- and the others with

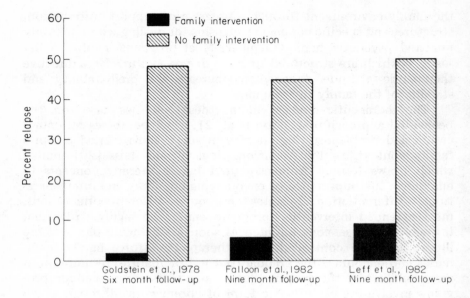

Figure 1. Relapse rates from three studies (Goldstein et al [7], Falloon et al [8], Leff et al [9]) contrasting a family intervention program with the absence of such a program (all schizophrenic patients on continuous medication).

nine-month follow-up. Although no final report has appeared as yet from the Anderson-Hogarty trial, preliminary reports [20] indicate a comparable low rate of relapse (10 percent) in their family therapy condition.

Overall, the pattern is very dramatic as four out of four studies report that some form of extended family intervention, overlaid on a program of regular pharmacotherapy, can make a substantial contribution to the reduction of relapse in recently discharged schizophrenic patients, even with those who have been chronically ill for a number of years. Longer-term follow-ups are needed to establish the durability of these changes, as well as whether such programs impact upon social role functioning as well.

SOME UNRESOLVED ISSUES CONCERNING COMBINED FAMILY AND DRUG THERAPY PROGRAMS

It seems quite clear that some form of family intervention is a very effective part of a comprehensive aftercare program. However, given that the programs evaluated so far in controlled clinical trials vary widely in their format, it is hard to know what aspects of the family intervention are significantly related to relapse prevention. The Leff et al program did not involve the patient at all, and while some family sessions were held, they relied primarily on relatives' groups to reduce contact and the likelihood of high EE behaviors at home [22]. The other programs cited above do involve the patient and operate within the traditional mode of family sessions with individual family units. Yet, evidence to date suggests comparable rates of relapse for all studies. This raises the question of whether these diverse family intervention programs offer a highly organized program of family support or whether, in contrast, they offer specific interventions beyond family system support. Further research is needed concerning the impact of these diverse models of family intervention in order to evaluate the specificity of their mode of action. Only one study so far has addressed this issue, as the Leff et al study repeated the Camberwell Family Interview (the instrument used to assess expressed emotion) before and after therapy for experimental and control subjects. Their family intervention program was found to reduce high EE attitudes in most cases, as compared with control subjects, and where attitude change had occurred, relapse was unlikely.

While there are no sharp differences to date in relapse rates, variations in family intervention programs may relate to the longer-term criterion of improvement in patient social functioning. Obviously, reducing the likelihood of relapse is a critical goal, but given the notoriously poor results to date in the rehabilitation of schizophrenic patients, evidence that any particular type of family intervention leads to improvement in social role performance would be very significant. Both the Falloon et al and Anderson-Hogarty programs have longer-term (two years) follow-ups built into them, and hopefully can provide data on these important issues.

Another issue that has not been addressed in recent controlled trials involving family and drug therapy relates to interactions between drug dose level and family intervention. The earlier study by the author [7] investigated this issue and found superior results when family therapy cases were maintained on the higher drug dose for the six-week controlled trial. However, this is a very brief period of both drug and family therapy, and more recent programs extend for a much longer period. Therefore, we still do not know whether an effective program of family intervention permits a reduction in drug dosage level, if not initially at least at some point during the first year of aftercare treatment. However, there are suggestions in the recently completed study by Falloon et al [8] that patients in the family therapy condition took their oral phenothiazine medication more regularly and were maintained at a lower dose level than patients in individual, supportive therapy. This suggests that it may be possible to reduce medication in combination with a longer-term family intervention program which lasts from nine months to a year after hospitalization for an episode of schizophrenia.

It would be very timely to investigate whether an effective program of family intervention can facilitate the use of a "targeted" medication program, in which patients are maintained at minimal or no drug status until prodromal signs of the disorder are evident, at which time therapeutic drug levels are utilized.

An interesting model to be tested in controlled clinical trials is whether an inverse relationship exists between the duration and intensity of a family intervention program and the dose level of maintenance pharmacotherapy. It could be hypothesized that a brief, crisis approach ("low-dose" family intervention) requires a higher maintenance drug dose level while an extended family program ("high-dose" family intervention) may permit a lower maintenance drug dose either initially or after the period of family treatment. Given the noxious side effects of phenothiazine drugs and the risk of tardive dyskinesia, any evidence that a systematic and organized family intervention program can permit a reduction in drug dose levels would be very significant and should be actively explored.

REFERENCES

1. Glick I, Hargreaves W, Raskin M, et al: Short versus long hospitalization. II. Results for schizophrenic inpatients. *Am. J Psychiatry* 132:385–390, 1975
2. Falloon IRH, Boyd JL, McGill CW, et al: Family management training in the community care of schizophrenia. In *New Developments in Interventions with Families of Schizophrenics*, edited by Goldstein MJ. San Francisco: Jossey-Bass, 1981
3. Hogarty GE, Schooler NR, Ulrich R, et al: Fluphenazine and social therapy in the aftercare of schizophrenic patients. *Arch Gen Psychiatry* 36:1283–1294, 1979
4. Kane JM, Rifkin A, Woerner M, Reardon G: Low dose neuroleptics in outpatient schizophrenics, *Psychopharmacol Bull* 18:20–21, 1982
5. Brown GW, Birley JLT, Wing JF: Influences of family life on the course of schizophrenic disorders: a replication. *Br J Psychiatry* 121:241–258, 1972
6. Vaughn CE, Leff JP: The influence of family and social factors on the course of psychiatric illness: a comparison of schizophrenic and depressed neurotic patients. *Br J Psychiatry* 129:125–137, 1976

7. Goldstein MJ, Rodnick EH, Evans JR, et al: Drug and family therapy in the aftercare of acute schizophrenics. *Arch Gen Psychiatry* 35:1169-1177, 1978
8. Falloon IRH, Boyd JL, McGill CW, et al: Family management in the prevention of exacerbations of schizophrenia: a controlled study. *N Engl J Med* 306:1437-1440, 1982
9. Leff J, Kuipers L., Berkowitz R, et al: A controlled trial of social intervention in the families of schizophrenia patients. *Br J Psychiatry* 141:121-134, 1982
10. Kane JM, Rifkin A, Quitkin F, et al: Fluphenazine vs placebo in patients with remitted, acute first episode schizophrenia. *Arch Gen Psychiatry* 39: 71-73, 1982
11. Marder SR, van Kammen DP, Docherty JP, et al: Predicting drug-free improvement in schizophrenic psychosis. *Arch Gen Psychiatry* 36:1080-1085, 1979
12. Huber G: Reine defekt syndrome und basisstadien endogener Psychogen. *Fortschr Neurol Psychiatr Ihver Grezvzgebiete* 34:409-421, 1966
13. Carpenter WT, Stephens JR, Rey AC, Hanlon TE, Heinrichs DW: Early intervention vs continuous pharmacotherapy of schizophrenia. *Psychopharmacol Bull* 18:21-22, 1982
14. Heinrichs DW, Carpenter WT Jr: The coordination of family therapy with other treatment modalities for schizophrenia. In *Family Therapy in Schizophrenia*, edited by McFarlane WR. New York: Guilford Press, 1983
15. Herz M, Melville C: Relapse in Schizophrenia. *Am J Psychiatry* 137:801-805, 1980
16. Nuechterlein KH: Developmental Processes in Schizophrenics Disorders. NIMH sponsored research grant MH30911, 1983
17. Anderson CM, Meisel SS, Houpt JL: Training former patients as task group leaders. *Int J Group Psychother* 25:32-45, 1975
18. Anderson C, Hogarty G, Reiss D: Family treatment of adult schizophrenic patients: a psychoeducational approach. *Schizophr Bull* 6:490-505, 1980
19. Goldstein MJ (ed): *New Developments in Interventions with Families of Schizophrenics*. San Francisco: Jossey-Bass, 1981
20. Anderson CM, Hogarty G, Reiss DJ: The psychoeducational family treatment of schizophrenia. In *New Developments in Interventions with Families of Schizophrenics*, edited by Goldstein MJ. San Francisco: Jossey-Bass, 1981
21. Vaugh C, Leff JP: The measurement of expressed emotion in the families of psychiatric patients. *Br J Soc Clin Psychol* 15:157-165, 1976
22. Berkowitz R, Kuipers M, Eberlin-Fries, et al: Lowering expressed emotion in relatives of schizophrenic patients. In *New Developments in Interventions with Families of Schizophrenics*, edited by Goldstein MJ. San Francisco: Jossey-Bass, 1981

CHAPTER 10

Agoraphobia: Behavioral Therapy and Pharmacotherapy

Matig R. Mavissakalian

Recent years have witnessed a surge of clinical research in agoraphobia and the development of effective behavioral and pharmacological treatments for this disorder [1-4]. These advances, in turn, have elucidated certain aspects of the nature of agoraphobia and have begun to suggest a rationale for combining pharmacotherapy and behavior therapy in the treatment of this complex disorder. Before discussing an integrated behavioral-pharmacological approach to the treatment of agoraphobia, therefore, a brief review of the disorder and the individual treatment modalities seems warranted.

Agoraphobia has been traditionally viewed as a phobic disorder because fears and avoidance behavior predominate in the clinical picture [5,6]. This view is reflected in the current Diagnostic and Statistical Manual of Mental Disorders [7] which requires the following two positive criteria for a diagnosis of agoraphobia: (1) the individual has marked fear of, and thus avoids being alone or in public places from which escape might be difficult or help not available in case of sudden incapacitation (eg, crowds, tunnels, bridges, public transportation), and (2) there is increasing constriction of normal activities until these fears or avoidance behavior dominate the individual's life. At its most severe, the condition renders the patient totally helpless and dependent on others for even the simplest of ventures outside the home. In less severe cases or stages of the disorder, however, patients can go out alone within a "secure" zone encompassing the immediate neighborhood or a few miles but cannot venture beyond these limits.

Several clinical, phenomenological, and psychophysiological differences have been noted between agoraphobia and simple phobias which call into question their common classification under phobias [8]. Indeed, a critical review by Hallam [9] suggested that agoraphobia could be more accurately considered a variant of anxiety neurosis and Goldstein and Chambless [10] identified the central fear of agoraphobia as the "fear of fear" which underscored the internal origin of the fear and its closeness to anxiety. Thus, on closer examination, most if not all patients reveal their essential fear of panicking, losing control, and consequently becoming physically, mentally, or socially anihilated (eg, "I am afraid I will have a heart attack and die;" "I am afraid I will faint and embarrass myself;" "I am afraid I will lose my mind and be hospitalized in a mental institution"). It is not surprising, therefore, that agoraphobics also have a fear of being alone, even in their own home, and that they only feel relatively secure in the company of trusted people.

Current conceptualizations of agoraphobia have thus emphasized the anxiety and panic components of the disorder [11]. This is supported by the chronically elevated background anxiety as well as the commonly experienced spontaneous (nonphobic) panic attacks of agoraphobic patients, and is reflected by the classification of agoraphobia under anxiety disorders and the introduction of the subgroup of agoraphobia with panic attacks in DSM-III. Thus, a hierarchical organization of the classification of anxiety disorders is implied whereby both panic and generalized anxiety disorders are encompassed by agoraphobia. Agoraphobia, then, can be justifiably construed as a complex anxiety disorder with elements of generalized anxiety, panic, and phobic anxiety and avoidance. The relationship of these dimensions is not yet fully understood, but the fact that behavioral treatments which target primarily phobic avoidance and antidepressants which target panic attacks have been found clinically effective in agoraphobia underscores the central importance of both dimensions in this disorder.

The clinical usefulness of antidepressant medications in the treatment of agoraphobia has, in addition, underscored the close yet elusive relationship between agoraphobia and depressive disorder. This multifaceted relationship includes (1) the onset of agoraphobia and panic disorder in the context of stressful life events and the frequently observed depressive symptomatology in agoraphobics, (2) the worsening of agoraphobia during depressive episodes, (3) the relatively high incidence of premorbid and emergent agoraphobia in major depressive disorder, (4) a high incidence of primary depression in agoraphobia as well as a high prevalence of depression and alcoholism in the first degree relatives of agoraphobics. Similarly, it has been shown that one half of anxiety neurotics develop secondary depression and that the majority of panic disordered patients give evidence of primary major depression [12-14]. Although this has led to questioning the nosological status of agoraphobia, the weight of the evidence as well as the temporal consistence of the agoraphobic syndrome strongly suggest that depression and agoraphobia are independent disorders but that agoraphobia (and anxiety disorders in general) may present liability to depressive disorder [15,16]. Clearly, more research is needed to elucidate the relationship of anxiety and depressive disorders. The degree of overlap, however, underscores the importance of assessing depression and mood changes in agoraphobia.

BEHAVIORAL TREATMENTS

Behavioral treatments have been rooted in experimental psychology and learning theory. The operant conditioning paradigm conceives of symptoms as freely emitted behaviors that produce and in turn are affected by environmental consequences. Accordingly, the major goal in the treatment of phobias (eg, to decrease avoidance behavior or to increase approach behavior) can be accomplished by reinforcing approach behavior or by removing all reinforcers for avoidance behavior. The classical conditioning theory, on the other hand, emphasizes both phobic anxiety and avoidance behavior and therefore is commonly known as the two factor theory. It conceptualizes phobic anxiety as a conditioned response to the phobic situation, escape from which is maintained through negative reinforcement (eg, anxiety reduction). Successful avoidance of the situation, on the other hand, conserves the anxiety and perpetuates the phobia [8].

Extensive research with behavioral methods aiming at the reduction of phobic anxiety and avoidance has revealed that successful treatments all share a common denominator, namely, exposure to feared stimuli [2,8]. Although at first it was thought that treatments should be initiated in imagination (eg, systematic desensitization or implosion) and then followed by exposure to the real phobic situation, recent studies have shown that the imaginal phase of treatment can be bypassed in most instances. As for the in vivo exposure, two methods seem equally viable. The first consists of gradually approximating the most feared situation by practicing exposure in incremental steps. For example, in the case of claustrophobia, the patient is instructed to enter an enclosed space and to remain there until he/she feels undue anxiety, at which time he is allowed to come out only to return to the situation and try to remain there a little longer. Feedback and praise (social reinforcement) often accompany this method, which is known as reinforced practice [17].

The other and more commonly utilized method of exposure is called prolonged in vivo exposure, based on the findings that given sufficient time, phobic anxiety declines (eg, habituation to a repetitive stimulus takes place) [18]. In this procedure commonly known as flooding patients confront phobic situations but, unlike reinforced practice, they are not allowed to escape when they become more anxious, rather they are encouraged to remain in the situation until their anxiety declines to comfortable levels and their urge to escape from it abates. Usually anxiety starts declining from its peak after 15 to 20 minutes of exposure which is continued for a total of 60 to 90 minutes [19].

In the literature, "exposed treatment" usually refers to prolonged exposure, but there is evidence that reinforced practice and prolonged exposure may be equally effective in the treatment of agoraphobia. Furthermore, the realization that what patients do between sessions is crucial for the success of treatment has led to greater reliance on self-directed in vivo exposure treatments. Indeed, Mathews and colleagues [2] have designed a treatment program which essentially hinges on providing patients therapeutic rationale and instructions for self-directed exposure (programmed practice) and which has shown promising results with agoraphobics. In addition, they have prepared manuals for patients and their spouses, which describe in detail the rationale and practice of self-directed exposure, and thus can reduce time spent in direct contact with the therapist.

In clinical practice, however, both methods of exposure could be utilized. Even in treatment utilizing prolonged exposure, a hierarchical approach proceeding from the least to the most fearful situation is often advisable, and it is not unusual for the therapist or a trusted surrogate to accompany patients in their first attempts at prolonged exposure. Similarly, benzodiazepines could be used as an aid to practice earlier on in treatment. Thus, recent reviews of the literature indicate that behavioral treatments based on exposure yield marked improvement in 60 to 70 percent of agoraphobic patients and that these gains are maintained over extended follow-up periods [20].

ANTIDEPRESSANTS

The rationale for the pharmacotherapy of agoraphobia, on the other hand, rests on clinical and experimental observations of the antipanic effect of antidepressants [11]. Indeed, both the MAO inhibitors (phenelzine) and tricyclics (imipramine) have been the subject of extensive investigations showing that they can be effective in the treatment of agoraphobia [3,4]. Although improvement rates are quite similar to those observed with behavioral treatments, a major difference with pharmacological treatments is the high relapse (approximately 25 percent) rates after cessation of the drug. Drop-out rates are also somewhat higher with pharmacotherapy and could be due to the reluctance of most agoraphobics to take pills. Furthermore, a particular oversensitivity characterized by insomnia, jitteriness, irritability, etc has been observed in one fifth of agoraphobics taking even small doses of imipramine. Recommended dosages are within the antidepressant range, although dose–response relationships have not been clearly established in the case of agoraphobia [21].

Furthermore, whereas there is general agreement in regard to the common mechanism inherent in behavioral treatments (eg, exposure/ habituation), the mechanisms underlying the antiphobic effect of antidepressants have not been elucidated. Since fear of panic is a central phenomenon in agoraphobia, and since patients do not seem to distinguish between their experience of spontaneous attacks and panic provoked by phobic situations, it is plausable to assume that successful control or suppression of spontaneous panic attacks can eliminate their potential to sensitize, reinforce, and maintain phobic anxiety and thus secondarily lead to reduction of avoidance. However, the relationship between the antipanic, antidepressant, and antiphobic effects of antidepressants is still puzzling.

The most common question asked has been whether antidepressants possess antipanic-antiphobic effects independent of their well-known antidepressant properties. The majority of workers have thus noted that initial levels of depression make no difference in outcome or even that higher scores of depression are associated with poorer outcome on several measures. These observations have suggested that the drugs' antipanic and antiphobic effects may not be mediated through their antidepressant effect, although a recent critical review of the literature has led Marks [22] to conclude that antidepressants "do not act reliably in the absence of dysphoria." Interestingly, McNair and Kahn [23] have observed that the antiphobic and antidepressant effects of imipramine may be related, whereas the drug's antipanic effect may be independent. It should be noted, however, that clinically, antidepressants have a global patholytic effect on mood (eg, depression, anxiety, and panic) and this, coupled with the high degree of correlations between symptom ratings, presents a major hurdle to the assessment of differential drug effects by symptom ratings alone [21].

Another major difficulty in assessing whether antidepressants have specific antiphobic effect is due to the use of support, encouragement, and even systematic instructions for in vivo exposure within most pharmacological trials [21]. Indeed, in a recent study with chronic agoraphobics treated with systematic in vivo exposure, Marks et al [24] failed to find any significant additional therapeutic effects due to imipramine. To date, the literature, with one exception, fails to provide an accurate assessment of the antiphobic effects of drugs proper. The exception is the 2×2 factorial study reported by Solyom et al [25] comparing the relative and combined effectiveness of exposure and phenelzine in the treatment of 40 agoraphobics and social phobics. Their results, based solely on specific measures of phobia, revealed that phenelzine and placebo were equally ineffective while exposure alone was found to be the active threapeutic ingredient.

To summarize, therefore, although the clinical usefulness of antidepressants in agoraphobia ia unquestionable, their mechanism of action is not clear. Clinically, drugs have a global patholytic effect on mood with some suggestion of a specific antipanic effect. However, whether they have a specific antiphobic effect or if reduction of avoidance behavior automatically follows improvement in mood is not known. Exposure treatments, on the other hand, effectively reduce phobic anxiety and avoidance. Thus, two treatments have been delineated, the one targeting the mood dimension and the other the behavioral dimension of agoraphobia, and it is but a small inferential leap to suggest that their combination would be clinically advantageous.

CONTROLLED STUDIES

In planning our investigation of the relative and combined effectiveness of behavioral and pharmacological treatments of agoraphobia, we established stringent methodological controls rendering all treatment conditions equivalent in all aspects except for the specific treatments being tested [26]. Thus, all patients in all treatment conditions were given the same rationale for treatment and spent the same amount of time in therapy and in contact with therapists. Furthermore, they all received drugs, 50 percent being randomly assigned to imipramine (up tp 200 mg) and the rest to double-blind placebo. In addition, they were all instructed to practice self-directed prolonged in vivo exposure between sessions. Thus, the control condition (C) was a powerful combination of all non-specific treatment factors and of programmed practice with experimental treatment groups in addition receiving either imipramine (I), therapist-assisted in vivo flooding (F), or a combination of imipramine-flooding (IF). The essential therapeutic question investigated in this study, therefore, was whether or not the addition fo pharmacotherapy and/or therapist-assisted exposure would enhance the known therapeutic effectiveness of the most basic and cost-efficient method of treating agoraphobics (eg, providing information and instructions for patients on how to treat themselves).

Another major aim of the study was to assess differential patterns of change across different symptom domains in the behavioral and mood dimensions of agoraphobia. Thus, a comprehensive assessment battery was developed which included self and clinician ratings of phobias, panic, anxiety, and depression, as well as behavioral avoidance tests. Finally, all patients were asked to keep a behavioral diary recording their daily out-of-the-home experiences. The diary data yeilded information on the frequency of outings, their duration, peak anxiety levels during these outings, and whether outings were practice or just part of the patient's routine. Practice was defined as an outing undertaken soley for the purposes of conducting prolonged in vivo exposure.

Before summarizing the outcome results, it would be informative to describe the treatment conditions in some detail. Treatment for all patients consisted of 12 weekly sessions. At each session they saw a psychiatrist individually, who adjusted drug dosage and met a clinical psychologist in groups of eight for 90 minutes of flooding in vivo or discussion. All patients were provided with the same rationale, emphasizing habitual avoidance as the main factor maintaining their fears and prolonged in vivo exposure/habituation as the method of choice in reducing and eliminating their fears. The importance of practicing exposure on their own was strongly and repeatedly emphasized and patients were told that whatever additional treatment or combinations thereof they may receive (eg, drugs, flooding, discussion) were intended to facilitate their effort at self-directed practices.

In this study, therefore, the use of drugs was adjunctive. One tablet of imipramine (25 mg) or placebo was inititated and the dose increased by 25 mg increments every second day, until a tolerable maintenance dose or a maximum of 200 mg/day was reached. The average maximal dose achieved with imipramine and placebo was 125 mg (SD = 66.6) and 6.5 tablets (SD = 2.3), respectively.

In the flooding condition, patients accompanied the therapist and assistants to the center of town or a large shopping mall in the hospital van. Once there, each patient was encouraged to leave the group and, either alone or with the help of the therapist at first, to enter individual stores or walk in crowded areas. The principle of prolonged exposure was strictly applied and patients were dissuaded from escaping the particular situation which they entered. Rather, they were encouraged to remain in these situations until their anxiety and urge to escape abated. Thus, treatment was individualized and tailored to each patient's need and pace of progress. The group discussions elaborated the behavioral rationale and instructions and reviewed in detail each patient's difficulties with exposure practice or reinforced gains made in the previous week. Although group members praised each other's achievements, the focus was on individual problems which the therapist addressed by making practical suggestions and selecting appropriate target activities for their next week's practice.

The outcome results (2×2 ANCOVAS) of 49 patients who completed the 12 week experimental phase IF = 12, I = 14, F = 12, and C = 11 revealed significant treatment effects on central measures

Table 1. 2×2 Analyses of Covariance Between Combined
Imipramine-Flooding, Imipramine, Flooding, and
Control Treatment Conditions

Major Dependent Measures at Postassessment	Main Effects F-Ratio	Medication Effects F-Ratio	Flooding Effects F-Ratio	Interaction Effects F-Ratio
GAS	4.83[†]	8.06[†]	2.77*	<1
FQ-T	3.36*	2.70	4.76*	1.52
FQ-AG	4.05*	3.03*	5.58*	1.52
PAA	3.26*	2.40	4.79*	2.91
BDI	3.31*	6.62[†]	<1	2.04
S-SUDS	3.23*	1.65	5.09*	2.43

*<0.05
†<0.01
Adapted from Mavissakalian and Michaelson: *Psychopharmacotherapy Bulletin* 1983: 19(1):117.

of agoraphobia [27]. As can be seen in Table 1, significant flooding effects were found on: (1) a five-point clinician rating Global Assessment of Severity (GAS), (2) the total fear score (FQ-T) and the agoraphobia sub-score (FQ-AG) of the Fear Questionnaire [28], (3) a nine-point clinical scale of Phobic Anxiety and Avoidance (PAA), and (4) measures of Subjective Units of Discomfort (S-SUDS) assessed on a nine-point analogue scale in the course of a standardized behavioral performance test. It can also be seen that in addition to GAS and FQ-AG, imipramine had a significant antidepressant effect as measured by the Beck Depression Inventory (BDI) [29]. Significant interaction effects between flooding and imipramine were not present.

To assess the clinical significance of these findings, patients were classified as high endstate functioning (HEF) and low endstate functioning (LEF), depending on whether they met three or four (HEF) or zero to two (LEF) of the following four criteria: (1) a score of 2 or less on the GAS (2 = mild condition and symptoms not interfering with normal work or social activities), (2) a score of 2 or less on a nine-point patient-rated scale of severity SRS (2 = slightly disturbing but not really disabling), (3) a score of 2 or less on the PAA representing the mean of five individual major phobic situations (2 = slight anxiety and hesitation to enter but rare avoidance), and (4) completing both behavioral performance tests with minimal or no anxiety. The first test (S-BAT) consisted of walking alone in an urban congested center over a 0.4 mile course and the second test (I-BAT) consisted of entering and remaining for at least five minutes in five idiosyncratically selected phobic situations (eg, church, large store, restaurant, bank, bus ride, etc.). At posttreatment, the proportion of patients meeting HEF was 73 percent in IF, 77 percent in I, 73 percent in F, and 33 percent in C conditions (X^2 = 5.4, 3 df; p = 0.14). Considered together, the three active treatments were significantly superior to the control (X^2 = 5.34; p = 0.02).

These results indicate that imipramine, flooding, and their combined treatments enhanced the therapeutic effectiveness of programmed practice to a statistically and clinically significant degree. However, these and additional analyses revealed that these three treatments did not differ at posttreatment, suggesting not only absence of additive or synergistic effect but equivalence between imipramine and flooding. Since all patients received behavioral instructions, the possibility was entertained that the potentiating effect of imipramine and flooding may have been due to increased practice in the more effective treatments [30]. However, analysis of the diary data did not show significant differences in frequency and duration of practice among the four groups. Nor did the groups differ significantly on nonpractice outings. The only major difference between the three experimental conditions and the controls, as well as HEF and LEF patients, was that subjective anxiety experienced during outings in general and practice in particular was significantly lower in the more effective treatments and in the HEF patients. This discrepancy between behavioral and subjective diary measures was paralleled by the results of Newman-Keuls analysis at posttreatment which revealed that the four treatment conditions did not differ on the two behavioral performance measures but that the control condition was significantly inferior in terms of clinical outcome measures and subjective anxiety experienced during the behavioral tests.

Figure 1 illustrates and compares differential patterns and rates of change between imipramine and flooding groups (n = 17 in each) across representative domains of psychopathology [31]. Univariate analyses of covariance, using the pretreatment measure as the covariate, were utilized to assess between group differences at the fourth, eighth, and twelfth weeks of treatment and at posttreatment. At the fourth week, imipramine effected significantly greater improvement (p <0.05) on measures of depression (BDI, Zung Depression Scale) and on Panic (0 to 8 patient-rated scale of "frequency and intensity of panic attacks, palpitations, breathlessness, sweating or trembling which you have had for no obvious reason during the past three days"), while flooding achieved significantly greater gains on S-BAT. Imipramine continued to effect significantly greater improvement on Panic, BDI, and GAS at week 8 and on measures of depression at week 12. At the posttreatment assessment there were no significant differences between the two groups on any measure except for BDI in favor of imipramine. It should be noted however, that BDI scores in both groups were below 9, which is not clinically significant. These results demonstrate that imipramine and flooding are equally effective in treating agoraphobia despite the early superiority of imipramine's effect on mood and the suggested specificity of flooding to reduce phobic avoidance.

If it is not through increased amount of practice, how do imipramine and flooding enhance the therapeutic effectiveness of programmed practice? We do not have clear answers to this question although some hypothetical ideas can be proposed at this time. It has been recognized that many processes other than exposure may determine fear reduction [32]. Among the cognitive factors, the development of a sense of mastery over the phobic situation (eg, self-efficacy) may be crucial [33]. It is possible, therefore, that the demonstration of habituation under the more reassuring circumstances created by the therapist's presence (in the flooding condition) may have induced a more positive cognitive set vis-a-vis practice and fostered greater self-efficacy early in treatment. Indeed, Marks et al [20] report that most of their patients did not require more than two supervised exposure sessions before they felt confident to conduct their own exposure treatment.

As to imipramine, it is quite possible that the drug's generalized patholytic effects on mood may have rendered practice more therapeutic by enhancing the process of habituation. There is theoretical and empirical evidence that high levels of arousal (eg, anxiety) and adverse mood (eg, dysphoria) can impede habituation [34,35]. Indeed, recent evidence suggests that depression, at least in the sense of severe dysphoric mood, can adversely affect habituation of fears in obsessive compulsive patients [36]. Perhaps imipramine's antipanic effect also minimizes the possibility of escape during exposure, and thus fosters prolonged exposure and habituation. Although this remains to be tested, evidence from studies with lactate-induced anxiety suggests that imipramine and MAO inhibitors can block spontaneous as well as provoked panic [37-39]. Furthermore, the ameliorative effect of imipramine on mood and panic as

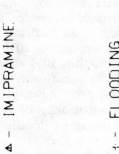

△ — IMIPRAMINE

+ — FLOODING

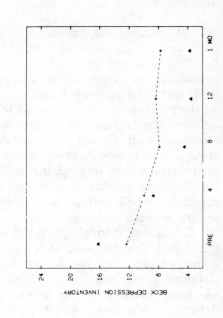

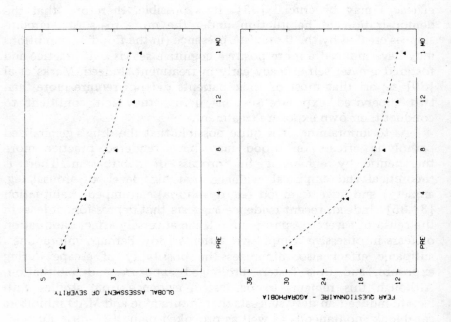

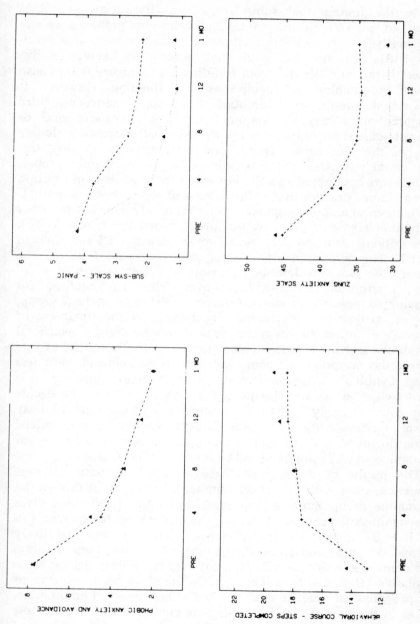

Figure 1. Measures of agoraphobia, anxiety, panic, and depression at pretreatment, four, eight, and 12 weeks of treatment and at posttreatment (one month) across imipramine and flooding conditions.

well as the finding that subjective anxiety during an equivalent amount of in vivo exposure practice and behavioral performance was significantly lower with imipramine are consistant with this possibility [30]. Still, our data show that patients are likely to derive greater therapeutic benefit from self-directed exposure if they also received imipramine or therapist-assisted flooding. However, it appears that, given a certain amount of exposure practice, one third of agoraphobics may not require additional pharmacological or therapist-assisted treatments. Since by design all patients, including those in the imipramine group, practiced exposure in vivo, this study could not assess the antiphobic effect of imipramine proper. We therefore conducted a small pilot study to assess the contribution of programmed practice to the effectiveness of pharmacotherapy [40].

Eighteen agoraphobic patients were randomly assigned to either imipramine (I) or imipramine plus programmed practice (I + BT). Three patients dropped out, leaving seven patients in I and eight in I + BT. The administration of drug was open and followed the gradual dose build-up described previously. Patients in the I + BT group, in addition, met individually with a clinical psychologist for programmed practice as described above. Patients in the I group, however, saw only a psychiatrist specializing in the treatment of depressive disorders. In this group, patients were not given behavioral instructions and the sole rationale offered was the beneficial effects of the drugs on mood and panic and their known clinical usefulness in agoraphobia. Questions relating to outings typically met with "Well, you are the best judge for that . . .", "You can decide when you feel ready." Thus, the treatment approximated the busy clinical practice of prescribing a medication known for its beneficial effects on mood and panic. The average maintenance daily dose of imipramine was 125 mg (range 50 to 200 mg) in both groups.

The results at the end of three months of treatment were interesting, even with this small number of patients. Although the imipramine group improved on most measures of outcome, there were significantly greater changes, primarily on phobic measures in the I + BT group. Group differences, however, were relatively minimal on panic and anxiety measures. Of course, these findings need controlled replication studies, but they tentatively suggest some antiphobic effect due to imipramine. On the other hand, it is evident that programmed practice enhances the effectiveness of imipramine, just as in the previous study imipramine enhanced the effectiveness of programmed practice. The mutual potentiation of the effects of imipramine and exposure suggests that in most instances both mood and behavioral dimensions of agoraphobia need focal treatment. On the other hand, it is clear that a considerable percentage of agoraphobics may be successfully treated with either imipramine alone or programmed practice alone. In these cases it would appear that breaking the vicious cycle at either the panic end or the avoidance end may be sufficient to lead to a reduction in both.

CONCEPTUAL AND PRACTICAL IMPLICATIONS

Despite the advances in therapeutics, our understanding of the etiology of agoraphobia has not progressed much beyond the well-known position of Freud that "generally there is a contribution of the two factors, the constitutional and the accidental" [41]. The genetic predisposition to neurotic illness has also been called anxiety proneness [42], one manifestation of which could be the increased autonomic activity and lability observed in anxiety neurotics and agoraphobics. Indeed, Lader and colleagues [43], in a series of psychophysiological studies, have demonstrated that anxiety neurotics and agoraphobics have elevated basal arousal levels and that they habituate more slowly than normal subjects. Furthermore, the physiological model of phobic anxiety and habituation proposed by Lader and Mathews [34] postulate that level of arousal (anxiety) is an important determinant of habituation: "a critical level of arousal would be predicted above which a repetitive stimulus would not be accompanied by any habituation; instead, level of arousal would become higher with each successive stimulus producing a positive feedback mechanism." In clinical practice, this positive feedback mechanism can be translated into panic and it can be suggested that the constitutional hyperaroused state of agoraphobics impedes the process of habituation and makes them more vulnerable to panic. Interestingly, Klein has also hypothesized a pathologically lowered central threshold in the production of panic attacks [11].

Bowlby's work and the notion of separation anxiety have recently attracted much attention vis-a-vis agoraphobia [11]. Furthermore, interesting parallels between the anxious behavior of humans and subhuman primates have been noted [44]. Of great interest is the development of a lasting tendency to react with fear and/or depression to subsequent separations and environmental changes in animals separated from their mothers during infancy. Of equal interest in this context is that these vulnerable animals have difficulty adjusting to new situations and characteristically take longer than control subjects before becoming fully engaged in the new environment. Finally, it appears that individuals subjected to repeated separations come to anticipate such separations and respond anxiously to any sign (eg, "threat") of imminent separations. Perhaps then, in addition to the genetic predisposition to panic, the vulnerability acquired by separation also contributes to the development of agoraphobia. The condition is likely to be particularly severe and chronic if the constitutional vulnerability to panic is complemented by the acquired proclivity to perceive stressful and even novel situations as threats.

Obstensibly, the major, if not only, difference between agoraphobia and panic disorder is the degree of behavioral avoidance. Our conceptualization of the nature of avoidance behavior therefore will determine the view of panic disorder and agoraphobia as either the same or separate disorders. In my view, the avoidance behavior of agoraphobics is nothing more than the natural extension of the tendency, clearly seen in panic disordered patients, to take precautionary measures to either prevent or minimize subsequent panic attacks. It is not at all surprising, therefore, that this would lead to avoidance of certain situations in which they expect to feel panicky. This would imply that the so-called spontaneous panic attacks or panic experienced in the phobic situation may be similar processes.

Thus, it is interesting that in our study, panic responded markedly and equally, albeit more slowly, to flooding than to imipramine. Similarly, panic attacks respond dramatically to paradoxical intention, a cognitive behavioral strategy (see later). Furthermore, there is now recent evidence showing that imipramine can significantly reduce phobic anxiety induced by exposure in addition to so-called spontaneous panic attacks or panic induced by lactate infusion [45]. This would suggest the use of caution in attributing an exclusive etiological treatment status to pharmacotherapy which purportedly would treat the core problem of "endogenous anxiety." It may be misleading therefore to label panic attacks as endogenous and phobic anxiety as exogenous simply because the provoking agent in the former eludes us or has not been thoroughly explored. Rather, it may be more accurate to conceptualize phobic anxiety provoked by exposure to phobic situations and panic attacks whether the source of provocation be chemical (lactate or isoprotonol infusion), physiologic (exercise), or still undetected (spontaneous?) as similar processes in agoraphobia.

Although the literature suggests a distinction between panic attacks experienced in phobic situations and the so-called spontaneous panic attacks of agoraphobics, the patients themselves do not differentiate between them. Furthermore, it is extremely difficult to tease out what is "spontaneous" and what is phobic in patients who are afraid of a multitude of situations and who become anxious even at the thought or prospect of an outing. In our center we therefore developed a conservative operationalized criteria for spontaneous panic attack as panic experienced at home without apparent external provocation. Even with this conservative measure, the majority of agoraphobics, nearly 70 percent, reported experiencing spontaneous panic attacks during the past week which suggests that it would be safe to assume that panic attacks are an integral part of the agoraphobic syndrome. It may therefore be justified to conceptualize panic disorder and agoraphobia as the same disorder. The puzzling question, of course, is why some panic-disordered patients do not develop agoraphobic avoidance. Alternative explanations for the origin of fears are offered by psychoanalytical and conditioning theories, neither of which is entirely satisfactory. Furthermore, a recent twin study [46] suggests that genetic factors don't play an important part in the strength and content of agoraphobic (separation) fears. Separation theory on the other hand, can explain the development of a generalized avoidant attitude. Maybe the difference between panic disorder and agoraphobia is one of severity, or, put another way, of degree of biological (genetic) or acquired (separation) vulnerability. At present, however, we must accept the inevitability of the accidental in the development of agoraphobic fears.

As was discussed earlier however, learning theory provides a parsimonious and valid explanation of the maintenance of avoidance behavior. Furthermore, with habitual avoidance the opportunity to reality test and habituate are lost, hence, the preservation of anxiety (eg, anticipatory anxiety). Also lost, according to Bandura, will be the opportunity to cope with the anxiety response, develop a sense of mastery and, thus, improve self-efficacy. Indeed, recent studies show a high degree of correlation between perceived self-efficacy, anticipatory anxiety, and avoidance [47]. It is exactly because of this self-perpetuating nature and its effect on self-efficacy and anticipatory anxiety, that exposure is a crucial element in the treatment of agoraphobia, and, I would venture to say, of panic disorder.

Anticipatory anxiety, as its name denotes, refers to the future occurrence of an event. As such, it has an attitudinal component, which can perhaps be best described as low self-efficacy, and usual psychophysiological components of anxiety, such as when the patient imagines himself or herself being in and coping poorly with the phobic situation. Anticipatory anxiety almost always also complicates the experience of panic as evidenced by the ubiquitous tendency to catastrophize (eg, the fear of fainting, of embarrassment, of heart attack, or of losing one's mind, etc). Moreover, it can itself become the source of a panic attack as when the concomitant psychophysiological distress becomes its own focus, leading to a positive feedback mechanism, ie, mild anxiety symptoms → anxious anticipation of panic → more intense anxiety → anticipation of dreaded consequences of panic → further increases of anxiety etc.

This scenario is the basis of a cognitive behavioral approach originated by Frankl [48] for the treatment of agoraphobia and panic attacks. Frankl further observes that in addition to excessive attention, excessive intention may also be pathogenic:

> Thus, we see an interesting parallel in that anticipatory anxiety brings about precisely what the patient fears, while excessive intention, as well as excessive self-observation with regard to one's own functioning, makes this functioning impossible. It is upon this two-fold fact that logotherapy bases the technique known as paradoxical intention. For instance, when a phobic patient is afraid that something will happen to him, the logotherapist encourages him to intend or wish for, even if only for a second, precisely what he fears (p. 146).

He goes on to explain that:

> This procedure is based on the fact that, according to logo-therapeutic teaching, the pathogenesis in phobias and obsessive compulsive neuroses is partially due to the increase of anxieties and compulsions caused by the endeavor to avoid or fight them. A phobic person usually tries to avoid the situation in which his anxiety arises, while the obsessive compulsive tries to suppress and thus to fight his threatening ideas. In either case the result is a strengthening of the symptom. Conversely, if we succeed in bringing the patient to the point when he ceases to flee from, or to fight his symptoms, but on the contrary, even exaggerates them, then we may observe that the symptoms diminish and that the patient is no longer haunted by them (p. 147).

In essence, therefore, paradoxical intention instructs the patients to take advantage of every opportunity to feel anxious and to try hard to panic. The emphasis on nonavoidance (exposure) of specific situations as well as the physiological and cognitive aspects of the experience of panic can be easily seen. It is therefore essentially addressed to the anticipatory anxiety of a phobic reaction before exposure and the anticipatory anxiety of panic during exposure and, as such, equates the treatment of phobias with that of panic. In addition, what paradoxical intention does is to change an overall avoidant attitude and eliminate self-defeating struggle with symptoms.

Struggle with symptoms, although the hallmark of compulsive behavior, is not infrequent in agoraphobia and panic. Indeed, recent conceptualizations of compulsive behavior suggest a functional equivalence between the better known compulsive washing or checking behaviors and all efforts cognitive or otherwise, to neutralize or reduce obsessions or the anxiety discomfort associated with them [49]. It should also be noted that compulsive behavior preserves obsessions much in the same way as avoidance behavior preserves phobic anxiety. The specific instructions to exaggerate symptoms of anxiety and their consequences therefore provide an alternative cognitive strategy in counteracting habitual cognitive patterns to either distract or relax oneself.

Thus, it can be easily seen how the frequent cognitive manuevers engaged by agoraphobics and panic disordered patients to distract themselves from the experience of anxiety or to compulsively attempt to neutralize or reduce the anxiety, for instance, with self-relaxation or the ingestion of tranquilizers, can be countered by the therapeutic instructions to focus on the symptoms of anxiety and paradoxically intend their exaggeration. From Frankl's theoretical vantage point however, "The purpose, to put it simply, is to enable the patient to develop a sense of detachment toward his neurosis by laughing at it" (p. 147). Thus, he advocates that paradoxical intention be carried out "in as humorous a setting as possible." The interjection of humor to paradoxical intention, however, is not contrived and has usually two sources. The first is the patient's insight into the futility and silliness of trying to induce or control a primarily physiological (autonomous) process such as anxiety. Second, it may be inherent in the paradoxical exaggeration of symptoms and feared consequences: "Die at least three times a day of a heart attack". "Show them what a wonderful passer outer you are". "I will show the world how to tremble". "I hope these folks know how to swim because I really intend to flood this room with my sweat."

Undoubtedly, paradoxical intention is a complex procedure involving several ingredients. Of interest is that it underscores the similarities between phobic anxiety and so-called spontaneous panic and emphasizes the crucial nature of anticipatory anxiety in both. It also provides a conceptual bridge between in vivo exposure and cognitive exposure emphasizing the importance of both behavioral nonavoidance and the development of a nonavoidant attitude. Finally, its perception of anxiety as primarily a physiological autonomic process conforms rather well to the habituation model of anxiety. The aim of the behavioral treatments, therefore, would be to eliminate the secondary elaborations and complications which prevent the natural process of habituation from taking place. In the case of agoraphobia, this would clearly include fostering nonavoidance of actual situations in which panic is experienced. In the treatment of panic, however, secondary complications involve more tacit cognitive maneuvers such as efforts to distract, suppress, or neutralize the experience of panic. It is clear, therefore, that paradoxical intention does not differentiate between its approach to phobic anxiety and panic.

Although systematic controlled studies of the effectiveness of paradoxical intention are lacking, the literature is replete with anecdotal reports of its effectiveness in the treatment of agoraphobia and panic. In my practice, I have found it to be an extremely useful strategy in treating patients with panic. In addition, a recent study in our center showed paradoxical intention combined with instructions for self-directed in vivo practice to be an effective treatment for agoraphobics [50]. However, perhaps its greatest merit is the reminder that in the treatment of agoraphobia and panic attacks, all components of the syndrome, namely, behavioral and cognitive avoidance, anticipatory anxiety, as well as phobic anxiety and panic, need therapeutic attention and that perhaps lasting improvement could not be achieved without changes in the patient's overall attitude.

The need to consider simultaneous treatment of all the components of the syndromes under discussion is suggested by the growing realization that despite their close relationships, they may be independent. Thus, phobic anxiety has come to be recognized as formed of three essential component response systems, namely, the subjective, the physiological, and the behavioral, which can covary or vary inversely or vary independently [51]. Furthermore, clinical observations provide some support of the relative independence of the panic/phobic anxiety and the avoidance/anticipatory anxiety components of agoraphobia. For example, with the pharmacological treatments, anticipatory anxiety and avoidance may persist despite successful reduction of panic/phobic anxiety. In addition, there are many agoraphobics, who after years of greater handicap and near total avoidance, manage to enter several previously avoided situations but continue to pay the price of undue discomfort and anxiety despite consistent exposure. Instances of desynchrony between these components therefore suggest that neither treatments specifically aimed at panic/phobic anxiety reduction, nor one relying solely on eliminating avoidance, can be expected to generalize across systems. However, synchronous changes with exposure do certainly occur when physiological and cognitive conditions are conducive to habituation. Similarly, it is plausible to suggest that because the primary aim of agoraphobics is to engage in hitherto avoided activities, imipramine may render even unstructured occasional exposures therapeutic by preventing the development of panic and, hence, premature escape from exposure. Furthermore, the antipanic effect of antidepressants may help patients tolerate the anxiety response without resorting to frantic efforts to neutralize it or to distraction during exposure, thus enhancing habituation. Clearly, a combined pharmacological/exposure approach would maximize the changes of synchronous and, hence, more complete improvement in agoraphobia and panic disorder. Furthermore, greater attention on the cognitive and tacit avoidance behaviors, and thus, anticipatory anxiety, is likely to reduce the problem of residual fear in the treatment of agoraphobia and probably may reduce relapse rates.

TREATMENT STRATEGY

In closing, let us attempt practical suggestions for an integrated approach to the treatment of agoraphobia. Consideration of the complex nature of this condition, which encompasses behavioral, mood, and cognitive dimensions, suggests that treatment planning should be based on the multidimensional functional analysis of each patient. Clearly, when clinical depression and/or severe handicapping panic attacks are present, they would indicate the use of antidepressants in their own right.

However, the literature clearly indicates, and our results confirm, that the majority of agoraphobics do not require antidepressants'

ameliorative effect on mood. Furthermore, it appears that at least
one third of patients given therapeutic rationale and instructions can
effectively treat themselves without therapist-aided exposure or
medications. Similarly, as mentioned earlier, I have found paradoxical intention to be an extremely effective strategy in the treatment
of panic attacks to the point that the majority of patients do not
require antidepressants. Therefore, based on the general premise that
the clinician's aim is to provide efficacious and cost-efficient treatment, as well as the realization that to date, except for early
improvement in treatment, none of the clinical or demographic
variables provide reliable prognostication, programmed practice in
addition to paradoxical intention seems an appropriate starting
point. In those patients who improve, unnecessary and costly treatment such as antidepressants or therapist-aided flooding would have
been avoided.

However, in those patients who do not improve or show only
minimal improvement after one month of treatment, the clinician,
probably depending on his or her background, would have a choice
between antidepressants or therapist-assisted flooding, which appear
to be equally efficacious when used adjunctively with self-directed
exposure. Our data furthermore indicate that combining in vivo
flooding and antidepressants may not be necessary in most cases.
In addition, the suggested approach would have the advantage of
rallying the patient's resource in his or her treatment and of
minimizing attribution of success to a pill or a therapist whose role
would be clearly defined as facilitating the patient's effort at
self-treatment.

Clinicians often see patients who are either unwilling or unable at
first to engage in self-directed practice. In these cases, a few therapist-
assisted in vivo exposure sessions, with the goal of teaching the
correct procedure of exposure as well as demonstrating the process
of habituation, may be sufficient to motivate the patient to pursue
treatment with self-directed exposure. However, when persuasion
fails to get the patient to the point of attempting exposure, and/or
the patient does not get the hang of paradoxical intention, the behavioral therapist may resort to a course of imaginal exposure treatments with either systematic desensitization or implosion with the
aim of reducing anxiety-provoked by the thought of being in phobic
situations (technically, anticipatory anxiety as discussed earlier). An
alternative approach could be to address directly the panic attacks
with antidepressants which, as discussed earlier, would be tantamount
to reducing phobic anxiety. Clearly, the majority of patients will

improve with this combined behavioral and pharmacological approach although a small number of patients will not. More research is required for the elucidation of individual characteristics which increase the risks of failure. As mentioned, cognitive and attitudinal factors, including personality structure, may be extremely important in such cases, necessitating treatment in their own right. Similarly, therapeutic attention to interpersonal and particularly marital maladjustment may be an important determinant of outcome [52].

ACKNOWLEDGMENT

This work was supported in part by the NIMH Grant MH-34177.

REFERENCES

1. Mavissakalian M, Barlow DH (eds): *Phobia: Psychological and Pharmacological Treatment*. New York: Guilford Press, 1981
2. Mathews AM, Gelder MG, Johston DW: *Agoraphobia: Nature and Treatment*. New York: Guilford Press, 1981
3. Mavissakalian M: Pharmacological treatment of anxiety disorders. *J Clin Psychiatry* 43:487–491, 1982
4. Sheehan DV, Ballenger J, Jacobsen G: Treatment of endogenous anxiety with phobic, hysterical, and hypochondriacal symptoms. *Arch Gen Psychiatry* 37:51–59, 1980
5. Snaith RPA: A clinical investigation of phobias. *Br J Psychiatry* 114:673–679, 1968
6. Marks IM: *Fears and Phobias*. London: Heinemann, 1969
7. *Diagnostic and Statistical Manual of Mental Disorders* (DSM-III), 3rd ed. Washington, DC: American Psychiatric Association, 1980
8. Mavissakalian M, Barlow DH: Phobia: An overview. In *Phobia: Psychological and Pharmacological Treatment*, edited by Mavissakalian M, Barlow DH. New York: Guilford Press, 1981
9. Hallam RS: Agoraphobia: a critical review of the concept. *Br J Psychiatry* 133:314–319, 1978
10. Goldstein AJ, Chambless DL: A reanalysis of agoraphobia. *Behav Ther* 9:47–59, 1978
11. Klein DF: Anxiety reconceptualized. In *Anxiety: New Research and Changing Concepts*, edited by Klein DF, Rabkin JG. New York: Raven Press, 1981
12. Mavissakalian M: Agoraphobia : The problem of treatment. *Behav Ther* 5:173–175, 1982
13. Dealy RS, Ishiki DM, Avery DH, Wilson LG, Dunner DL: Secondary depression in anxiety disorders. *Compr Psychiatry* 22:612–618, 1981
14. Raskin M, Peeke HVS, Dickman W, Pinsker H: Panic and generalized anxiety disorders. *Arch Gen Psychiatry* 39:687–689, 1982

15. Klerman GL: Anxiety and depression. In *Handbook of Studies on Depression*, edited by Burrows GD. New York: Exerpta Medica, 1977
16. Roth M, Mountjoy CQ: The distinction between anxiety states and depressive disorders. In *Handbook of Affective Disorders*, edited by Paykel ES. New York: Guilford Press, 1982
17. Leitenberg H: *Handbook of Behavior Modification and Behavior Therapy*. Englewood Cliffs, NJ, Prentice-Hall, 1976
18. Marks I: *Cure and Care of Neuroses:Therory and Practice of Behavioral Psychotherapy*. New York: John Wiley, 1981
19. Marshall WL, Gauthier J, Agordon A: The current of flooding therapy. *Prog Behav Mod* 7:205-275, 1979
20. Jansson L, Ost L: Behavioral treatments for agoraphobia: An evaluative review. *Clin Psychol Rev* 2:322-336, 1982
21. Mavissakalian M: Antidepressants in the treatment of agoraphobia and obsessive-compulsive disorder. *Compr Psychiatry* 24:278-284, 1983
22. Marks IM: Are there anticompulsive or antiphobic drugs? Review of the evidence. *Br J Psychiatry* 143:338-347, 1983
23. McNair DM, Kahn RJ: Imipramine compared with a benzodiazepine for agoraphobia. In *Anxiety: New Research and Changing Concepts*, edited by Klein DF, Rabkin JG. New York Raven Press, 1981
24. Marks IM, Gray S, Cohen D, et al: Imipramine and brief therapist-aided exposure in agoraphobics having self-exposure homework. *Arch Gen Psychiatry* 40:153-162, 1983
25. Solyom C, Solyom L, LaPierre Y, et al: Phenelzine and exposure in the treatment of phobias. *Biol Psychiatry* 3:239-247, 1981
26. Mavissakalian M, Michelson L: Agoraphobia: behavioral and pharmacological treatments. Preliminary outcome and process findings. *Psychopharmacol Bull* 18:91-103, 1982
27. Mavissakalian M, Michelson L: Agoraphobia: behavioral and pharmacological treatment (n = 49). *Psychopharmacol Bull* 19:116-118, 1983
28. Marks IM, Mathews AM: Brief standard self-rating for phobic patients. *Behav Res Ther* 17:263-267, 1979
29. Beck AT, Ward CH, Mendelson M, Mock J, Erbaugh J: An inventory for measuring depression. *Arch Gen Psychiatry* 4:53-63, 1961
30. Mavissakalian M. Michelson L: The role of self-directed practice in behavioral and pharmacological treatments of agoraphobia. *Behav Ther* 14:506-519, 1983
31. Mavissakalian M, Michelson L: Agoraphobia: behavioral and pharmacological treatment, submitted for publication
32. Rachman S: Emotional processing. *Behav Res Ther* 18:51-60, 1980
33. Bandura A: Self-efficacy: towards a unifying theory of behavioral change. *Psychol Rev* 84:191-215, 1977
34. Lader MH, Mathews AM: Physiological model of phobic anxiety and desensitization. *Behav Res Ther* 6:411-421, 1968
35. Foa EB: Failure in treating obsessive-compulsives. *Behav Res Ther* 17:169-176, 1979
36. Foa EB, Steketee GS, Ozarow BJ: Behavior therapy with obsessive-compulsives: from theory to treatment. In *Obsessive Compulsive Disorder: Psychological and Pharmacological Treatment*, edited by Mavissakalian M, Turner S, Michelson L. New York: Plenum Press, in press

37. Appleby IL, Klein DF, Sachar EJ, et al: Biochemical indices of lactate-induced panic: a preliminary report. In *Anxiety: New Research and Changing Concepts*, edited by Klein DF, Rabkin J. New York: Raven Press, 1981

38. Kelly D, Mitchell-Heggs N, Sherman D: Anxiety in the effects of sodium lactate assessed clinically and physiologically. *Br J Psychiatry* 119:468-470, 1971

39. Liebowitz MR, Klein DF: Agoraphobia: clinical features, pathophysiology and treatment. In *Agoraphobia: Multiple Perspectives on Theory and Treatment*, edited by Chambless DL, Goldstein AJ. New York: John Wiley, 1982

40. Mavissakalian M, Michelson L, Dealy RS: Pharmacologic treatment of agoraphobia: imipramine vs imipramine with programmed practice. *Br J Psychiatry* 143:348-355, 1983

41. Freud S: Analysis terminable and interminable. In *Collected Papers*, vol. 5. New York: Basic Books, 1959 (originally published 1937)

42. Shields J: Genetic factors in neurosis. In *Research in Neurosis*, edited by van Praag HM. New York: SP Medical and Scientific Books, 1978

43. Lader MH: Physiological research in anxiety. In *Research in Neurosis*, edited by van Praag HM. New York: SP Medical and Scientific Books, 1978

44. Suomi SJ, Kraemer GW, Baysinger CM, DeLizo RD: Inherited and experiential factors associated with individual differences in anxious behavior displayed by Rhesus monkeys. (n *Anxiety: New Research and Changing Concepts*, edited by Klein DF and Rabkin J. New York: Raven Press, 1981

45. Ko GN, Elsworth JD, Roth RH, et al: Panic-induced elevation of plasma MHPG levels in phobic-anxious patients. *Arch Gen Psychiatry* 40:425-430, 1983

46. Torgersen S: The nature and origin of common phobic fears. *Br J Psychiatry* 134:343-351, 1979

47. Bandura A, Reese L, Adams N: Microanalysis of action and fear arousal as a function of differential levels of perceived self-efficacy. *J Pers Soc Psychol* 43:5-21, 1982

48. Frankl VE: *Psychotherapy and Existentialism*. New York: Simon and Schuster, 1967

49. Rachman S: The modification of obsessions: a new formulation. *Behav Res Ther* 15:437-443, 1976

50. Mavissakalian M, Michelson L, Greenwald D, Kornblith S, Greenwald M: Cognitive-behavioral treatment of agoraphobia: paradoxical intention vs self-statement training. *Behav Res Ther* 21:75-86, 1983

51. Rachman SJ: *Fear and Courage*. San Francisco: W. H. Freeman and Company, 1978

52. Chambless DL, Goldstein AJ (eds): *Agoraphobia: Multiple Perspectives on Theory and Treatment*. New York: John Wiley and Sons, 1982

CHAPTER 11

Anorexia Nervosa: Psychological Therapies and Pharmacotherapy

Elke D. Eckert and Katherine A. Halmi

Anorexia nervosa is best viewed as a heterogeneous disorder featuring multiple deficits in psychological, social, behavioral, and biological functioning. Treatment is therefore integrated and multifaceted; it must also be flexible since not all elements of treatment are equally relevant to each patient or to each phase of illness. Both physical and psychological aspects of the disorder must be considered; physical aspects have precedence when weight is low and anorectic behavior dominant, while psychological aspects have precedence when weight is normal and anorectic behavior is under control. This approach makes sense when one realizes that starvation itself produces abnormalities in cognition, emotionality, and physiological changes similar to those present in anorexia nervosa [1,2]. Treatment may last up to several years, and may require a combination of various psychotherapies, including behavior therapy and pharmacotherapy.

PSYCHOLOGICAL THERAPIES

Several psychological therapies have been advocated for anorexia nervosa. These include psychoanalytic [3], a special "fact finding" psychotherapy [4], simple supportive therapy [5], family therapy [6,7], cognitive therapy [8], and various behavior therapies. [9–12]. The effects of psychological treatments have not been adequately assessed. Most systematic assessments have involved behavior therapy; moreover, the only randomized controlled study done has evaluated the effectiveness of behavior therapy [13].

It is natural for behavior therapy to emerge as a treatment for this condition because anorexia nervosa can be viewed as an eating and weight phobia—eating or weight gain generates anxiety and failure to eat or weight loss serves to avoid anxiety. From this analysis two behavioral procedures are suggested: systematic desensitization to reduce anxiety and thus allow normal eating to emerge, and operant conditioning by using powerful reinforcers contingent on eating or weight gain, thus allowing anxiety to take care of itself. There are few reports describing systematic desensitization as treatment for anorectics and only one case report in which desensitization is used alone [9]. Operant conditioning has received more attention and systematic studies using behavior therapy have used selective positive reinforcements consisting of increased physical activity, visiting privileges, and social activities contingent on weight gain, and powerful negative reinforcements such as bed rest, isolation, or tube feeding for failure to gain weight [12].

Agras and associates [10], using applied behavior analysis in single case experiments, isolated four important variables contributing to control of weight gain in anorectic patients. Patients often eat in order to leave the hospital, an example of negative reinforcement. Positive reinforcement for weight gain is important but is maximally effective only when informational feedback to patients about weight and calorie intake is used in conjunction. The fourth variable is the amount of food served; the larger the amount served, the more is eaten. A combination of all four variables appears most effective.

Only one randomized controlled study has tested the efficacy of behavior therapy. This study, a large multi-center project, found no difference in weight gain between standard milieu treatment and the combination of standard milieu treatment and reinforcement of small increments of weight gain [13]. However, evidence indicates that the particular behavioral program used in this study was not maximally effective. The limited length of study time of 35 days may have been insufficient to demonstrate a significant treatment difference. The program did not use individualized reinforcements. Individual reinforcements may be more effective than constant reinforcers used in all patients. The schedule of reinforcements may be a significant factor. The program reinforced weight gain every five days rather than daily. One of the authors has shown, by utilizing both daily and delayed reinforcement programs consecutively in individual patients, that daily reinforcement is more effective for weight gain than delayed reinforcement [14].

Although no clear advantage has been demonstrated for behavior therapy, most if not all effective empirically based programs have incorporated behavioral techniques into their treatments even if they are not so identified. Likewise, effective behavioral programs also utilize other psychotherapies. Agras [15], in a recent literature review on behavior therapy in anorectics, found behavior therapy to be more efficient; that is, patients treated with behavior therapy (consisting of structured reinforcement for weight gain in a hospital setting) had an increased rate of weight gain compared with those treated with medical therapy (consisting of hospitalization often combined with confinement to bed, supervised eating, psycho- therapy, family therapy, and occasionally tube feeding) or with drug therapy. Given present concerns with cost-effectiveness, it seems prudent to utilize treatments that offer rapid results.

Principles of Psychotherapeutic Practice

There are four general treatment goals for an anorectic patient: (1) to gain and maintain weight, (2) to resume normal eating pat- terns, (3) to assess and treat relevant psychological issues in the patient, and (4) to educate families about the disorder by assessing the family's impact on maintaining the disorder and assisting them in developing methods to promote normal functioning of the patient. Before these treatment goals are discussed it is necessary to explain two basic principles of treatment.

1. Exposure and response prevention as principles of treatment for anorexia nervosa

Anorexia nervosa can be viewed, in part, as an anxiety-based dis- order explainable by learning theory. Regardless of the initial stim- ulus for dieting, eating or weight gain begin to generate anxiety, while not eating and weight loss serve to avoid anxiety. Behaviors such as taking laxatives and self-induced vomiting further reduce anxiety by preventing weight gain. In time, binge-eating, vomiting, and food faddism come to dominate the anorectic's life and usually begin to function autonomously from the original motivation for weight loss. Therefore, these food-related behaviors must be addressed specifically.

Because of these features, the illness has been compared with obsessive-compulsive [16] or phobic disorders [17]. It has been shown that a helpful treatment for obsessive-compulsive disorder involves exposure to the anxiety-producing stimuli and prevention of the compulsive rituals (response prevention) [18]. In phobic disorders, the essential therapeutic requirement is thought to be exposure to the phobic object [19]. However, there is some controversy concerning how precisely anorexia nervosa can be regarded as a phobic illness. Salkind [20] has argued against a precise association because he has found minimal skin conductance changes in anorectic patients to the presentation of a series of food and weight-related stimuli.

Rosen and Leitenberg [21] have described, in a study of a normal weight bulimic patient, that exposure and response-prevention were effective in eliminating binge-eating and vomiting, reducing anxiety after eating, and increasing food intake without vomiting.

Application of these treatment principles to anorexia nervosa requires exposure to the twin fears, eating and weight gain. We observe clinically that exposure to weight gain and normal eating is associated with gradual reduction of these fears. Preliminary reports have shown that psychological improvement does occur with weight gain [22, 23]. Further systematic studies specifying the extent of these changes are necessary. If this principle of treatment is accepted, several different approaches to treatment may be effective, provided the patient eats and gains weight. In practice these treatments may include "forced feedings," operant contingencies for eating or weight gain, or the presentation of structured diets in which the patient is persuaded to eat.

An extention of these principles involves using response prevention to treat anorectic "rituals" which have an anxiety-reducing function. These rituals include vomiting after meals, "food faddism," use of laxatives, compulsive exercising, and weighing frequently. Response prevention entails forced avoidance of these rituals, for example, not allowing access to laxatives and monitoring after meals to stop vomiting.

The precise approach to each patient is based on clinical judgment. In general, patients should retain as much control as possible as long as the desired result is achieved. However, patients who cannot or will not cooperate with the necessary "exposure" require external controls to in effect "force" the physiology back to normal since the starvation state induces neurotransmitter changes, hormonal changes, depression, and other biological changes. This external control is obviously more easily done in the hospital than in the outpatient clinic. If external controls are applied, especially in the hospital, it is imperative that gradual transfer of control back to the patient be accomplished before discharge. This means that if external controls such as structured diets, tube feeding, or operant contingency programs for weight gain are initially used, a patient should not be discharged before she resumes control over eating and weight. This resumption of control is usually done by a graded stepwise procedure. To discharge a patient before she has been able to accomplish this is an open invitation for relapse.

2. Weight gain, weight maintenance and the resumption of normal eating patterns

The treatment goals of gaining and maintaining weight and resuming normal eating patterns are best considered together. An attempt at outpatient treatment can be made. However, if hospitalized, a structured eating program and the use of behavioral contingencies on eating and weight gain are helpful. Such a program will be described.

A. Medical stabilization phase The first few days of hospitalization serve two purposes: medical stabilization and assessment of the external controls needed. The expectation is that the patient will at least maintain her weight during the first few days. Further weight loss is not tolerated and leads to consequences which will be described.

The anorectic behaviors needing correction are defined through observation and discussion with the patient. This leads to judgments concerning what external controls will be necessary. Hospitalization alone sometimes provides enough structure for patients to establish control which includes stopping the abnormal behaviors such as binge-eating and vomiting. If these behaviors continue, they are addressed using response prevention techniques such as mealtime monitoring by nursing staff in order to prevent binge-eating, the hoarding of foods, and vomiting. This monitoring may be necessary for one or two hours after meals, including accompanying patients to the bathroom to prevent vomiting.

Since it is expected that no further weight loss will occur, and since the patient has probably already demonstrated that she needs external control due to failure at outpatient therapy, strict control of the diet is maintained by the staff during the stabilization phase. She is begun on a balanced diet of 1,500 calories per day in divided meals which she will be required to finish. This may include "feared" foods which she has systematically deleted from her diet, only foods not associated with extreme anxiety, or a nutritionally balanced liquid diet. A liquid diet is useful because some patients feel less anxious drinking their calories than eating them. It also allows them to avoid making decisions about which foods to eat. However, it is imperative that "feared" foods soon are systematically added since exposure to them is important. Not to do so would be to condone maintenance of anorectic behavior.

If the patient does not finish the food provided within a pre-scribed length of time, specific contingencies follow. For example, the next meal may be liquid. If that meal is not finished in the specified time, tube-feeding will take place. Given clear guidelines and strict application of the treatment plan, tube feeding is rarely needed. If tube fed once, most patients will not require it again. Intravenous feeding is rarely necessary and the necessity for hyper-alimentation is exceedingly rare.

B. Weight gain phase   A goal weight (or in reality a goal weight range as will be described later) is decided on; this should not be lower than the weight which will assure regaining menses [23]. This is often taken to be the lowest normal standard weight for age and height (Metropolitan Life Insurance Compant weight-height scale; pediatric growth chart). No negotiation is allowed on this. The patient is expected to gain an average of 0.5 pound per day. This is realistic and a safe rate of gain for most patients. In actual practice, we make a weight graph for the patient indicating the expected weight gain with a diagonal line. Operant contingencies for weight gain are used; these consist of a combination of individualized daily reinforcers plus a gradual expansion of off-ward privileges. The reinforcers are earned on any day that the patient's weight achieves or exceeds the expected minimum. If this fails, we sometimes change to an operant plan which requires that the patient remains isolated in her room for 24 hours if her weight falls below the expected weight for the day. This program involving isolation is very effective in promoting weight gain in most patients [14]. There are occasional patients who are socially withdrawn and prefer to isolate themselves in their rooms. For these patients it is better to make access to their rooms contingent on weight gain.

If a controlled diet is utilized, the guidelines mentioned earlier apply. Calorie content of provided food gradually increases to approximately 3,500 Kcal per day. This is generally enough to insure the required weight gain. Meals are given at prescribed times only. Measures to prevent vomiting and binge-eating may be used.

C. Weight maintenance phase As patients approach their goal weight, their anxiety may again increase at the prospect of being unable to either regulate or maintain weight. A period of weight maintenance lasting two to four weeks at "normal weight" before discharge may reassure the patient that she will not keep gaining and get "fat." We think that this period also helps to correct body image distortion, to solidify psychiatric gains, and to allow time for the physiological changes to stabilize. We find it best to change the goal to a range of weights once their goal weight has been attained. This range is usually 4 pounds: 2 pounds above and 2 pounds below the goal weight. Since some weight fluctuation is inevitable, keeping weight within a range is a more realistic goal, thus protecting against anxiety.

During weight maintenance, the external control on the diet will again vary depending on individual needs. The goal is to eat normally during this time and, if external controls are still applied, they must be gradually removed before discharge. If eating in various situations, such as restaurants, is a potential problem the patient may benefit from practice sessions. For example, staff may accompany the patient the first time she goes for an outing to a restaurant. Later she can practice eating in situations alone, with family members, and with others.

We normally continue using operant behavioral contingencies for maintaining weight during the maintenance phase. This involves daily off-ward privileges for the patient who remains within the goal range. These contingencies are removed before discharge to test her capacity to maintain weight on her own.

This maintenance period is intended to provide gradual transition to outpatient status. When it is clear that she is maintaining her weight, we encourage passes home for increasingly long intervals. This is useful because problems involved with transition to the home environment can be identified and addressed before discharge.

3. Assessment and treatment of psychological issues

A. Supportive treatment during weight gain phase (patient education) While weight is low and eating behaviors are very disordered, psychotherapy should mainly support efforts to modify eating behavior and gain weight.

First, patients are repeatedly educated about the effects of starvation and the physiological changes which can be expected as weight is regained. The anorectic's illogical thinking concerning weight and food issues is usually very engrained. A typical example of illogical thinking is the belief that within just a few days of eating normal meals the required weight will be gained. To counter this illogical idea, the actual process of what is involved in weight gain is conveyed. Patients are instructed that the starvation process slows the digestive system, increases the time necessary for gastric emptying, and causes constipation. The result is that they will feel "full" despite eating very little. Less often patients will feel hungry despite a large meal. This unnatural hunger may reinforce the anorectic's fear of "losing control." They are taught that this is an effect of starvation which will diminish with weight gain.

Weight gain is associated with physiological and anatomical changes which may be distressing. A straightforward approach to this is best. Patients are warned that as rapid weight gain occurs, the added weight may not be properly distributed. Redistribution may take a month of maintenance at normal weight. Weight gained will appear first on the trunk and face areas; this distribution produces an enlarged "tummy" and waist and a round face. This faulty distribution reinforces "feeling fat." Patients need to ignore these feelings temporarily.

B. Common psychological themes Once starvation is no longer a factor, weight gain has occurred, eating problems are under control, and fears of weight gain have diminished, significant psychotherapeutic issues rekindled by the return of overt signs of biological maturity become evident. Each patient has a unique set of problems, but there are common and recurring themes. These are a failure to acknowledge illness, disturbance in cognition, problems with separation and autonomy, poor psychosicial skills, a negative self-concept, and defective recognition and expression of certain affective states. Through a problem-oriented reeducative therapy, we focus on each specific problem and teach patients skills needed to facilitate normal thinking and functioning.

Failure to acknowledge illness: The failure of some anorectic patients to acknowledge illness, or "denial" of illness, is a frustrating and difficult problem. They may fail to acknowledge their thinness and to acknowledge hunger and fatigue. This "denial" is compounded by the pleasure they derive from being thin. In addition they interpret attention given their thinness as acknowledgement that being thin is desirable. No sure way to break through this impediment to treatment is available. However, various techniques involving confrontation, at times gentle and at times forceful, are helpful.

Straightforward confrontation of the thinness is not the most effective approach. More positive response may be obtained by a discussion of associated symptoms of the illness which the anorectic can agree are problems and which she may want to correct. These include symptoms starvation has produced: sleep disturbance, irritability, depression, preoccupation with food, and social alienation. Physicians often think that pointing out a dangerously low serum potassium level to a patient, resulting from vomiting, or diuretic or laxative abuse, should shock her into acknowledging the illness and cooperating with treatment. Such an approach is often ineffective. The reasons are probably multiple; one is that the patient does not feel the effect of the low serum potassium level in her body, and hence she disbelieves the doctor's pronouncement.

The anorectic illness may be thought of as an avoidance of life problems. Failure to acknowledge illness sometimes extends beyond the strictly anorectic issues to include psychological changes. "Denial" may serve a purpose: it may be the glue that holds a shattered self-esteem together. Hence, high levels of support must be available if the patient is to begin to acknowledge illness. Psychotherapy must focus painstakingly on the appeal for the patient to remain anorectic versus the fear and drawbacks of being at normal weight. The anorectic illness with its associated behaviors and its past, present, and future consequences must receive firm emphasis in treatment. Other anorectics, especially in groups, can often more effectively confront these issues than an individual therapist. They can also provide the necessary understanding and support to help patients accept their illness.

Disturbances in cognition: Disturbed cognition involves distortion of body image as well as the already described distortion in the areas of food and weight. Disturbed cognition may extend to other areas as well. For example, anorectic patients often exaggerate self-reference. They not only feel that other people watch every bite they put into their mouths and will notice every ounce of weight gain, but they also feel that they are the focal point of everyone's attention. These distortions are repeatedly "labelled" and corrected with cognitive confrontation [8]. Body distortion is brought to the patient's attention early in treatment [24]. The patient is told that during weight gain, she will probably continue to misperceive her body size because this misperception will constantly be reinforced by the physiological changes which will be occurring. She is told that she cannot trust her own perceptions in this area and must temporarily ignore these feelings.

Problems with separation and autonomy: Many authorities think that the anorectic illness begins when the individual fails to proceed normally toward independence. The illness may exaggerate dependent, immature, or regressed traits, often reinforced by family members. Independence is encouraged in therapy. One element in this is to teach the patient to distinguish her motivations from the expectations of others. This ability is an integral part of normal adolescent maturation.

Poor psychosocial skills: Many anorectic patients have major interpersonal problems and follow-up studies have shown they have high levels of social anxiety [25]. They are often described as shy and nonassertive. These difficulties are often present before the onset of illness, but they are certainly compounded by the disruption of normal social development associated with this illness. Assertiveness and social skills training can be invaluable.

Negative self-concept: Anorectic patients often have a negative self-concept. Starvation reinforces this self-concept because of the associated depression and increasing withdrawal and alienation. Also, the perfectionism and high expectations typical of anorectics are difficult standards to maintain and increase the likelihood of failure. Shy and nonassertive behavior adds to low self-esteem. Cognitive correction plus assertiveness and social skills training can help. However, low self-esteem may be an aspect of depression which may respond to drug treatment.

Defective recognition and expression of affective states: Certain affective expressions, especially anger, may not be recognized by anorectics or, if recognized, are inappropriately expressed (perhaps by not eating). Patients often think it inappropriate to feel and especially to express anger. They need to be taught to recognize, accept, and appropriately express feelings. Keeping a written journal about difficult interactions coupled with assertiveness training is helpful.

Teaching these skills can be accomplished in part in groups but each patient will have problems needing individual attention, at least initially. Some, especially those with a good premorbid adjustment, may require little while others will have greater difficulty facing the problems of adolescence and life in general. An ongoing open relationship with a therapist they can respect and trust, who can share experiences and be a role model, may be extremely important.

Education of families: If the patient is living at home, education of the family is important to the patient's recovery. Family members should be interviewed early to assess their concerns and to teach them about the course, prognosis, and treatment of anorexia nervosa. This often relieves guilt feelings and anxiety. Early contact with them is also important to obtain their help in engaging the patient in treatment, and to establish an alliance between family members and the therapeutic team so treatment efforts will not be sabotaged.

If a patient is hospitalized, the family should be seen or at least contacted weekly. Anorectic patients are notorious for their manipulations. This behavior springs from their anorectic fears as well as their poor interpersonal skills. For example, patients when first admitted to the hospital often complain about the therapeutic program, the food, the staff, or almost anything else. However, they may not direct their complaints to the staff but instead to family members. The family should be warned and instructed not to collude with patients by getting involved in these issues. They should instead refer the patient back to the treatment team. Family members are requested not to talk about weight and food issues with patients. They should leave those to the patient and the treatment team.

In outpatient treatment, the family and patient should attempt to agree on an approach to food and weight. Although generally the family should have little direct involvement in these matters except to support constructive efforts, there are exceptions. For example, after failing to gain weight on her own, one 14-year-old patient agreed to eat a specified diet only if her mother would serve it. She could or would not serve herself; she could not decide on portions, played and fussed with food, became increasingly anxious, and eventually did not eat. Having the mother serve was an acceptable initial step since weight gain was the first priority. It also accomplished the necessary exposure to normal eating we have described. Later, of course, the patient had to manage her own meals. Consistency, not rigidity, is emphasized to help relieve the confusion and anxiety surrounding eating. Limits on anorectic behavior within the family are warranted. Families must not let the anorectic illness dictate dietary habits or otherwise dominate the family life. For example, special low calorie diets offered in an attempt to stimulate food intake seldom get the anorectic to eat. Such measures only reinforce the illness. Other limits may be placed on binge-eating and vomiting by requiring payment for missing food and requiring that the bathroom be cleaned after vomiting.

It is also important that the treatment team understands the interrelationships within the family system. If necessary, this can wait until starvation is no longer a factor since it is difficult to focus on the interrelationships and problems within the family while the illness itself demands attention. It is also likely that relationships within the family will have changed in the emergency presented by the starving child. Faced with this, the family often reinforces the illness and the patient's dependency. It is vitally important that the family understands this and is helped to overcome it by promoting more autonomous functioning of the patient. The amount of help needed will vary from case to case. Some families will require only a few sessions while others will require prolonged therapy.

Despite hospitalization and other intensive attempts to help the family, some anorectic patients will do better in a long-term placement away from their home. Some more seriously ill patients may need a carefully chosen residential treatment center or day care center and halfway house which can continue to give appropriate attention to weight and food and otherwise encourage psychological development.

PHARMACOTHERAPY

There is a growing literature base concerning possible benefits of various pharmacotherapies in anorexia nervosa. However, like the psychological therapies, treatment effects have not been adequately assessed. Only a few systematic controlled studies have been reported.

Pharmacological interventions are best appreciated from understanding neuropharmacologic feeding regulatory mechanisms. These mechanisms are complex and not well understood. A brief discussion of what is known about them follows.

Feeding Regulatory Mechanisms

The hypothalamus is involved in the control of a variety of basic functions, including eating behavior. The medial hypothalamus acts as a "satiety center." Stimulation of this area in animals causes cessation of eating even when they should be hungry. Destruction of this area can cause aninals to overeat and become obese. The lateral hypothalamus in contrast, acts as a "feeding center," with stimulation of this area leading to eating behavior and destruction leading to cessation of eating and weight loss. These two areas appear to be linked by reciprocal inhibition [26].

Several neurotransmitter systems pass through and probably help regulate these areas [26]. An intact nigrostriatal dopamine pathway appears to be necessary for adequate feeding or for facilitation of the lateral hypothalamus. Lesioning this dopamine pathway can lead to hypophagia. Drugs augmenting dopamine, such as L-dopa, should facilitate eating. However, the relationship of dopamine to eating mechanisms is obviously not a simple one. Another theory speculates that increased dopaminergic activity is involved in anorexia nervosa and argues that dopamine blocking agents should be useful [27].

Serotonin appears to facilitate medial hypothalamic satiety [26]. Agents such as parachlorophenylaline, which depletes serotonin, increase eating behavior in animals. Serotonin antagonists such as cyproheptadine should therefore facilitate eating. Two controlled studies using this drug in the treatment of anorexia nervosa will be discussed later.

Adrenergic effects, involving norepinephrine and epinephrine, appear to have different effects depending on the site of action and whether or not beta or alpha-adrenergic functions are involved [28].

Other systems, such as the endogenous opiate system, also appear to be involved in appetite regulation. Circulating beta-endorphin levels are elevated in genetically obese mice [29] and also in obese humans [30]. Naloxone, the narcotic antagonist, can abolish overeating in the obese mice [29]. More recently, cholecystokinin, a peptide involved in digestive function, has been shown to have a neurotransmitter function which appears to suppress appetite in animals [31]. It is obvious that the more these feeding regulatory mechanisms are studied, the more complex they appear.

Review of Pharmacotherapy for Anorexia Nervosa

Many drugs have been reported to benefit patients with anorexia nervosa but most have not been tested in large systematic well-controlled studies. Case reports and open trial studies reporting benefits (usually weight gain) have involved the following drugs:

chlorpromazine with and without insulin, pimozide, imipramine, amitriptyline, lithium, chlorimipramine, tryptophan, cyproheptadine, L-dopa, naloxone, phenoxybenzamine, ACTH, and cortisone. Only some of these drugs will be discussed.

Chlorpromazine was the first drug used in treating anorectics. Used in doses ranging from 150 to 1,000 mg per day, this drug is reported to facilitate weight gain and shorten hospitalization [32]. It would be worthwhile to do a controlled study using chlorpromazine. Naloxone has been infused into anorexia nervosa patients to determine its effect on weight gain. Weight gain was calculated for periods before, during, and after use of the medication. Patients were reported to gain more weight during the time of drug infusion but since this was an open trial with no systematic methodology and patients were receiving antidepressant medication concurrently, no conclusions can be made [33]. Naloxone deserves more careful study regarding its effect on appetite regulation and weight control.

Patients with anorexia nervosa have been demonstrated to have abnormal gastric functioning, including delayed gastric emptying and decreased gastric fluid output. In a recent study metoclopramide, a dopamine blocker and properistaltic agent, was found to enhance gastric emptying and improve gastrointestinal symptoms of anorectic patients, including improved tolerance for eating and less postprandial epigastric pain, belching, vomiting, anorexia, and early satiety [34]. No adverse effects were noted.

Controlled studies have been done using chlorimipramine, lithium, pimozide, cyproheptadine, and amitriptyline. Chlorimipramine showed no advantage to weight gain over placebo in a small randomized controlled study, although the anorectic patients receiving it reported an increased appetite and tended toward improved weight maintenance after leaving the drug trial [35]. Lithium was found in one four-week double-blind placebo controlled trial involving 16 anorectic patients to be superior to placebo in effecting weight gain in weeks 3 and 4 of treatment [36]. The authors suggested caution concerning the use of lithium in these patients because of the possibility of rapid lithium toxicity caused by vomiting, laxative or diuretic abuse, or inadequate fluid intake. In a placebo-controlled crossover study using pimozide in the treatment of 18 anorectic patients, there was a suggestion that pimozide enhanced weight gain although the results were not statistically significant [37]. Pimozide had a marginal effect on anorectic attitudes in the same study.

Cyproheptadine is one of the most interesting and attractive drugs for the treatment of anorexia nervosa. It is an antihistamine with serotonin antagonist action and a chemical structure related to tricyclic antidepressants. Although marketed in this country as an antihistamine, the pharmaceutical company promotes it primarily as a weight-inducing agent for cattle. The drug has also been reported to promote weight gain in a variety of populations including asthmatic children, underweight adults, and patients with irritable bowel syndrome. Cyproheptadine has also been tried in the treatment of anorectic patients because of its effect on weight gain. However, in 1977, Vigersky and Loriaux [38] reported no significant difference in weight gain between cyproheptadine and placebo groups in an eight-week controlled study of 24 hospitalized anorectics.

The results of a multi-center randomized double-blind cooperative effort involving the treatment of 105 hospitalized anorectic patients with cyproheptadine or placebo were reported in 1979. The authors of this chapter were two of the investigators in this study. In a preliminary analysis of 81 patients, cyproheptadine was effective in inducing weight gain in a more severely ill subgroup of anorectics: those who (1) had a history of birth complications, (2) were more emaciated, and (3) had a history of prior outpatient treatment failure in terms of weight gain [39]. However, in the final analysis of 105 patients, the investigators were unable to detect a main effect of cyproheptadine on weight gain. This was perhaps due to the study design. According to this design the dose of cyproheptadine was gradually increased depending on weight gain with the result that few patients received the maximum dose of 32 mg per day. Those who did receive the maximal dose only received it a short time—for the last five days of the 35-day treatment. However, the investigators were able to establish cyproheptadine as a safe drug in anorectics, even at the maximal dose of 32 mg per day. There are no complicating side effects such as hypotension, increased cardiac irritability, and undesirable interactions with other drugs. Hence, it is an attractive drug for this frequently medically unstable patient group. Interestingly, cyproheptadine did have a significant effect on typical anorectic attitudes in this study [40]. It was associated with reduced preoccupation with a thin body ideal, reduced interest in food and cooking, increased heterosexual interest, and increased sociability. These results suggested that increase in the cyproheptadine dose as well as increase in duration of treatment might show a significant effect on weight gain as well as on improving anorectic attitudes.

Thus, the authors undertook a second collaborative study treating hospitalized anorectics with cyproheptadine utilizing larger doses and a longer treatment time.

In the same study the authors also decided to test the efficacy of another medication, amitriptyline. Evidence is accumulating for an association between affective disorder and eating disorders. Anorexia nervosa patients are often depressed before the onset of the anorectic illness and they may have increased risk for affective illness after the acute anorectic illness [41]. During the acute anorectic illness they show a variety of depressive symptoms including sleep disturbance, irritability, depressed affect, crying spells, and social withdrawal [22]. Additionally, there are biological indicators present in the acute anorectic illness which are also associated with depression, including dexamethasone nonsuppression [42], decreased urinary MHPG secretion [43], and impaired growth hormone response to L-Dopa [44]. Many clinicians have been using antidepressants in treating anorectics. A few open-trial studies have suggested amitriptyline to be effective in inducing weight gain and relieving dysphoria in these patients [45,46].

Hence, the authors thought that two drugs, cyproheptadine and amitriptyline, would be most interesting to evaluate in treatment of acute anorexia nervosa. Seventy-two such patients were treated in-hospital in randomized double-blind assignment to one of three drug treatments (32 mg of cyproheptadine, 160 mg of amitriptyline, or placebo). Treatment lasted until they reached normal weight or a maximum of 12 weeks. Patients gaining less than 2 kg after six weeks of drug treatment were considered treatment failures. Preliminary analysis of 57 cases in this study revealed that cyproheptadine, given in sufficiently high doses (32 mg per day), induced significantly more weight than placebo and, surprisingly, improved mood by reducing depression score ratings on the Hamilton Depression Scale [47]. Final analysis of the total sample of 72 patients is still underway.

COMBINING PHARMACOTHERAPY AND
PSYCHOLOGICAL THERAPIES

Psychological therapies are the mainstay of most treatment programs for anorexia nervosa. Only one controlled study has addressed the efficacy of combining psychological therapy and drugs. In the multi-center hospital study mentioned earlier, involving 105 anorectic patients at low weight treated randomly with either cyproheptadine or placebo, patients were also treated randomly with or without behavior therapy [13,39]. The four treatment groups in this study were: cyproheptadine and behavior therapy, cyproheptadine and no behavior therapy, placebo and behavior therapy, and placebo and no behavior therapy. Although an analysis of a possible additive or interactive effect of cyproheptadine and behavior therapy was never reported, this analysis was done. The results indicate that there was no advantage to weight gain in the cyproheptadine and behavior therapy group compared with the other three groups. No specific subgroups of patients emerged which gained more weight with a combination of these two therapies.

Although no research exists indicating benefits to combining pharmacotherapy with psychological therapies in anorectic patients, we empirically propose a theoretical framework and speculate on problems in combining these two treatment modalities.

Combining Treatments in the Acute Anorectic State

During the acute anorectic state, abnormalities in neurotransmitters, hormones, and other biological variables largely reflect starvation. Starvation must be reversed. Various behavioral methods assuring in-vivo exposure and response prevention to normalize weight and eating behavior are probably faster than nonbehavioral psychological therapies. If approached in the right manner these therapies are accepted by most patients. Characteristics such as "fear of getting fat" may be "nonendogenous" features of anorexia nervosa which may best respond to psychological methods such as exposure to the fear of weight gain by having patients gain weight and then maintain weight. Drugs may affect "endogenous" anorectic symptoms such as decreased gastric emptying time, hyperactivity, mood changes, obsessionality, sleep disturbance, and certain anorectic attitudes. We think that an approach which combines psychological techniques (mostly behavioral) and medication should be most effective at this acute phase of illness.

Until research can adequately examine these speculations, medications should be used as adjunctive treatment on an individualized basis. Cyproheptadine in high final doses (32 mg per day) appears helpful in facilitating weight gain and in reducing depressive symptoms, and appears safe despite the unstable physical condition of many acute anorectics. A starting dose of 4 mg three or four times per day is well tolerated and the dose can be rapidly increased. No complications have been observed with the medication and the only usual side effects are mild sedation and dry mouth.

Chlorpromazine may be useful for severely obsessional or highly anxious anorectics. It should be started in small doses of 10 to 40 mg a day since phenothiazines may aggravate hypotension and other cardiovascular problems seen in anorectics. The dose can be slowly increased depending on the response obtained.

Although depressive symptoms usually improve as weight is gained, amitriptyline and other antidepressants may be useful for significantly depressed anorectics. Pharmacologic treatment of depression at this phase of illness may allow greater energy and motivation to be applied to more strictly anorectic problems. These medications should also be started at small doses and increased with caution because of the possible aggravation of already existing cardiovascular instability associated with starvation. The most common side effects of the antidepressants are anticholinergic; they include dry mouth, sedation, tachycardia, and postural hypotension. The usual final dose for antidepressants such as amitriptyline or imipramine should not exceed 3.5 mg/kg/day to maintain a serum level between 150 and 250 mg/ml.

Gastrointestinal symptoms may be treated with medication. Metoclopramide, in a single 10 mg oral dose, may enhance gastric emptying and improve gastrointestinal symptoms such as bloating.

Poor patient drug compliance is an issue as some patients will refuse medications and some will agree to take them but will surreptitiously spit them out. Close patient monitoring with mouth checks after taking medication can often circumvent the latter situation. Blinder [48] has described an interesting approach utilizing a combination of behavioral contingencies and the use of medication. For a patient who disliked taking chlorpromazine, he made reduction of the dose given contingent on weight gain, thus using chlorpromazine as a negative reinforcer.

Combining Treatments in the Residual Anorectic State

Psychiatric reassessment should be done after weight gain when effects of starvation are eliminated. Residual psychiatric symptoms will have important treatment implications.

Clinicians who see many anorectic patients have recently noted an increased frequency of secondary anorectic illness. They are seeing more anorectics with primary diagnoses of personality disorders, affective disorder, anxiety disorders, or even schizophrenia who develop a typical anorectic illness secondarily.

The presence or absence of a personality disorder may best be decided only after weight gain since the starvation state may obscure correct evaluation. For example, starvation increases obsessive-compulsive thinking and behavior. After weight gain these character-istics should be improved. The remains of these characteristics may be an evident reflection of personality or an expression of depression requiring antidepressant medication. Anorectics frequently possess "borderline" personality traits during the starvation state. Our clinical experience indicates these traits improve with weight gain. Reassessment of patients having these traits after weight gain should consider the possibility of an affective disorder like cyclothymia or a bipolar II disorder which may respond to medication. Akiskal [49] has recently suggested that personality disorders such as borderline, cyclothymic, or even severe obsessives may be subclinical, "subsyn-dromic," or "subaffective" manifestations of affective disorders which may respond to lithium or antidepressants. (However, lithium is gen-erally contraindicated because of the possibility of lithium toxicity caused by vomiting, laxative or diuretic abuse, or inadequate fluid intake [50].)

There is practically no literature which addresses the use of medi-cations after weight gain in anorectic patients. Therefore, medica-tions must again be used according to individual indications. For example, patients with significant residual anxiety after weight gain, either associated with irrational ideas about weight and food intake or more generalized anxiety, may respond to medications such as cypro-heptadine or chlorpromazine. Although minor tranquilizers may also be effective in this regard, there is no literature concerning this. If minor tranquilizers are used, it must be with caution in patients with bulimia who as a group have a high addiction potential.

Antidepressants should receive strong consideration. Low self-esteem and problems with motivation and passivity may indicate the presence of depression, even though the patient's symptoms may not meet full diagnostic criteria for major depression. We often find that self-esteem and motivation are improved with antidepressants. Psychotherapy may then proceed more rapidly since patients will more readily try new experiences.

Some medications may worsen specific anorectic symptoms. For example, it has been suggested that amitriptyline may contribute to bulimic symptoms because it has been shown to produce carbohy-drate craving in a nonanorectic population [51]. Whether or not medications such as amitriptyline may be at risk in precipitating bulimia in some anorectic patients is a worthwhile research question since bulimic symptoms are common in these patients at follow-up. Some indirect evidence against this point of view exists in that both imipramine [52] and MAOI antidepressants [53] have recently been reported to significantly reduce the number and intensity of bulimic episodes in patients with the bulimia syndrome.

Other residual psychological problems after weight gain include issues of dependency, cognitive distortions, and social interactional problems. They are best treated with reeducative psychotherapy techniques using individual, group, and family therapy approaches, much as described earlier. Psychiatric assessment after weight gain should determine which of these treatment modalities are necessary.

Residual anorectic fears about food intake and weight control can continue to be addressed specifically using behavioral techniques. It may be important to continue in-vivo exposure to these pervasive anorectic "fears." At this phase of therapy, which will primarily be on an outpatient basis, this involves use of behavioral techniques which the patient can control and apply. These may include keeping a record of food intake, using structured meal plans, practicing "nonanorectic" eating, and using self-reinforcement for appropriate eating behavior or weight maintenance. The Eating Disorders Clinic at the University of Minnesota provides patients with a structured monitoring sheet on which to self-monitor meals and problem behaviors. Although not all patients will need such devices, these labelling and feedback procedures can help them feel better able to control their behavior.

These behavioral techniques can be utilized in either individual or group treatment. We have found groups helpful for anorectics who are motivated to improve. The role-modeling by recovering anorectics as well as the support and appropriate confrontation by the entire group can be powerful. Patients often remark later in treatment how important it was for them to have observed the improvement of others.

Treatment triangles involving psychiatrists, other medical specialists, and nonmedical psychotherapists are prevalent for anorectic patients because combined treatment approaches are often necessary. Psychiatrists or other medical specialists may assess the need for and prescribe medications and monitor the anorectic's physical status. At the same time, nonmedical psychotherapists may do individual, family, or group therapy. It is essential that professionals involved form an agreement about their respective responsibilities and how they will interact. Such an agreement is particularly necessary for anorectic patients who are often extremely difficult to manage and treat. A common view of psychopathology and treatment philosophy for the anorectic illness is best. Frequent contacts between the involved professionals are necessary. Treatment will run more smoothly and be more effective with adherence to a sound agreement.

CONCLUSIONS AND FUTURE DIRECTIONS

A combination of psychological therapies is the mainstay of most effective treatment programs for anorexia nervosa. Pharmacotherapy is utilized as adjunctive treatment based on individual need. The number of well-designed research studies testing efficacy of these treatments is amazingly small and practically no information is available concerning efficacy of combining psychotherapy and pharmacotherapy. This paucity of research is remarkable since anorexia nervosa is increasing in frequency and costs for treatment, which may take years, can be high.

Comparison of results in studies done is hampered by methodologic problems related primarily to inconsistencies in design and measurement procedures plus small sample size. The few well-controlled studies done have tested treatment efficacy of either pharmacotherapy and/or behavior therapy in short-term outcome of low-weight anorectics. Results of these studies indicate both pharmacologic therapy and operant behavioral techniques may be effective in improving weight gain. Additionally, drugs may improve associated symptoms.

Clearly, more and better controlled studies are necessary to test both short-term and long-term outcome. Studies of long-term outcome in part depend on the identification of effective short-term treatment.

It makes empirical sense to combine psychotherapy with pharmacotherapy in this difficult illness. However, before such combination treatments are evaluated, research should be aimed at identifying which components of the total treatment programs are effective for which components of the anorectic illness.

REFERENCES

1. Keys A, Brozek J, Henschel A, et al: *The Biology of Human Starvation.* Minneapolis: University of Minnesota Press, 1950
2. Schiele BC, Brozek J: Experimental neurosis resulting from semistarvation in man. *Psychosom Med* 10:31–50, 1948

3. Silverman J: Anorexia nervosa: clinical observations in a successful treatment program. *J Pediatr* 84:68-73, 1974
4. Bruch H: *Eating Disorders*. New York: Basic Books, 1973
5. Farquharson RF, Hyland HH: Anorexia nervosa: the course of 15 patients treated from 20 to 30 years previously. *Can Med Assoc J* 94:411-419, 1966
6. Minuchin S, Baker L, Rosman B, et al: A conceptual model of psychosocial illness in children: family organization and family therapy. *Arch Gen Psychiatry* 32:1031-1038, 1975
7. Selvini Palazzoli M: *Self-Starvation*. London: Chaucer Publishing, 1974
8. Garner DM, Bemis K: A cognitive-behavioral approach to anorexia nervosa. *Cogn Ther Res* 6:1-27, 1982
9. Hallsten EA Jr: Adolescent anorexia nervosa treated by desensitization. *Behav Res Ther* 3:87-91, 1965
10. Agras WS, Barlow DH, Chaplin NH, et al: Behavior modification of anorexia nervosa. *Arch Gen Psychiatry* 30:279-286, 1974
11. Azerrad J, Stafford RL: Restortation of eating behavior in anorexia nervosa through operant conditioning and environmental manipulation. *Behav Res Ther* 7:165-171, 1969
12. Halmi KA, Powers P, Cunningham S: Treatment of anorexia nervosa with behavior modification. *Arch Gen Psychiatry* 32:93-96, 1975
13. Eckert ED, Goldberg SC, Halmi KA, et al: Behavior therapy in anorexia nervosa. *Br J Psychiatry* 134:55-59, 1979
14. Eckert ED: Behavior modification in anorexia nervosa: a comparison of two reinforcement schedules. In *Anorexia Nervosa: Recent Developments in Research*, edited by Darby PL, Garfinkel PE, Garner DM, Coscina DV. New York: Allen R. Liss, 1983
15. Agras WS, Kraemer HC: The treatment of anorexia nervosa: do different treatments have different outcomes? In *Association for Research of Nervous and Mental Diseases*, Vol. 62, edited by Stunkard AJ, Stellor E. New York: Raven Press, 1983
16. Solyom L, Freeman RJ, Miles JE: A comparative psychometric study of anorexia nervosa and obsessive neurosis. *Can J Psychiatry* 27:282-286, 1982
17. Crisp AH: Anorexia nervosa: 'feeding disorder', 'nervous malnutrition', or 'weight phobia'? *World Rev Nutr Diet* 12:452-504, 1970
18. Steketee G, Foa EB, Grayson JB: Recent advances in the behavioral treatment of obsessive-compulsive disorder. *Arch Gen Psychiatry* 39:1365-1371, 1982
19. Klein DF, Zitrin CM, Woerner MG, et al: Treatment of phobias. II. Behavior therapy and supportive psychotherapy: are there any specific ingredients? *Arch Gen Psychiatry* 40:139-145, 1983
20. Salkind MR, Fincham J, Silverstone T: Is anorexia nervosa a phobic disorder? A psychophysiological enquiry. *Biol Psychiatry* 15:803-808, 1980
21. Rosen JC, Leitenberg HL: Bulimia nervosa: treatment with exposure and response prevention. *Behav Ther* 13:117-124, 1982
22. Eckert ED, Goldberg SC, Halmi KA, et al: Depression in anorexia nervosa. *Psychol Med* 12:115-122, 1982
23. Frisch RE: Food intake, fatness, and reproductive ability. In *Anorexia Nervosa*, edited by Vigersky R. New York: Raven Press, 1977
24. Slade PD, Russell GFM: Awareness of body dimensions in anorexia nervosa: cross-sectional and longitudinal studies. *Psychol Med* 3:118-199, 1973

25. Stonehill E, Crisp AH: Psychoneurotic characteristics of patients with anorexia nervosa before and after treatment and at follow-up 4-7 years later. *J Psychosom Res* 21:189-193, 1977
26. Hernandez L, Hoebel BG: Basic mechanisms of feeding and weight regulation. In *Obesity*, edited by Stunkard AJ. Philadelphia: WB Saunders, 1980
27. Barry VC, Klawans HL: On the role of dopamine in the pathophysiology of anorexia nervosa. *J Neural Transm* 38(2):107-122, 1976
28. Leibowitz SF: Identification of catecholamine receptor mechanisms in the perifornical lateral hypothalamus and their role in mediating amphetamine and L-Dopa anorexia. In *Central Mechanisms of Anorectic Drugs*, edited by Samanin R. New York: Raven Press, 1978
29. Margules D, Moisset B, Lewis M, et al: Beta-endorphin is associated with overeating in genetically obese mice (ob/ob) and rats (fa/fa). *Science* 202: 988-999, 1978
30. Givens JR, Wiedemann E, Andersson RN, et al: Beta-endorphin and beta-lipotropin plasma levels in hirsute women: correlation with body weight. *J Clin Endocrinol Metab* 50:975-976, 1980
31. Morely JE: The neuroendocrine control of appetite: the role of endogenous opiates, cholecystokinin, TRH, gamma-aminobutyric-acid and the diazepam receptor. *Life Sci* 27:355-368, 1980
32. Dally PJ, Sargant W: A new treatment of anorexia nervosa. *Br Med J* 1: 1770-1773, 1960
33. Moore R, Mills IH, Forster A: Naloxone in the treatment of anorexia nervosa: effect on weight gain and lipolysis. *J Roy Soc Med* 74:129-131, 1981
34. Saleh JW, Lebwohl P: Metoclopramide-induced gastric emptying in patients with anorexia nervosa. *Am J Gastroenterol* 74:127, 1980
35. Lacey JH, Crisp AH: Hunger, food intake and weight: the impact of clomipramine on a refeeding anorexia nervosa population. *Postgrad Med J* 56:79-85, 1980
36. Gross HA, Ebert MH, Faden VB, et al: A double-blind controlled trial of lithium carbonate in primary anorexia nervosa. *J Clin Psychopharmacol* 1:376-381, 1981
37. Vandereycken W, Pierloot R: Pimozide combined with behavior therapy in the short-term treatment of anorexia nervosa. *Acta Psychiatr Scand* 66:445-450, 1982
38. Vigersky FA, Loriaux DL: The effect of cyproheptadine in anorexia nervosa: a double-blind trial. In *Anorexia Nervosa*, edited by Vigersky R. New York: Raven Press, 1977
39. Goldberg SC, Halmi KA, Eckert ED, et al: Cyproheptadine in anorexia nervosa. *Br J Psychiatry* 134:67-70, 1979
40. Goldberg SC, Eckert ED, Halmi KA, et al: Effects of cyproheptadine on symptoms and attitudes in anorexia nervosa (letter). *Arch Gen Psychiatry* 30:1083, 1980
41. Cantwell PD, Sturzenberger SD, Burroughs J: Anorexia nervosa—an affective disorder? *Arch Gen Psychiatry* 34:1087-1093, 1977
42. Gerner RH, Gwirtsman HE: Abnormalities of dexamethasone suppression test and urinary MHPG in anorexia nervosa. *Am J Psychiatry* 138:650-653, 1981
43. Halmi KA, Dekirmenjian H, Davis JA, et al: Catecholamine metabolism in anorexia nervosa. *Arch Gen Psychiatry* 35:458-460, 1978

44. Halmi KA, Sherman BN: Prediction of treatment response in anorexia nervosa. In *Biological Psychiatry Today*, edited by Obiols J, Ballus C, Gonzalez E, et al. Amsterdam: North-Holland Biomedical Press, 1979

45. Needleman HL, Waber D: The use of amitriptyline in anorexia nervosa. In *Anorexia Nervosa*, edited by Vigersky R. New York: Raven Press, 1977

46. Mills I: Amitriptyline therapy in anorexia nervosa. *Lancet* II:687, 1976

47. Halmi KA, Eckert ED, Falk JR: Cyproheptadine, an antidepressant and weight-inducing drug for anorexia nervosa. *Psychopharmacol Bulletin* 19:103-105, 1983

48. Blinder BJ, Freeman DA, Stunkard AJ: Behavior therapy of anorexia nervosa: effectiveness of activity as a reinforcer of weight gain. *Am J Psychiatry* 126:77-82, 1970

49. Akiskal HS: Subaffective disorder: dysthymic cyclothymic, and bipolar II disorders in the 'borderline' realm. *Psychiatr Clin North Am* 4:25-36, 1981

50. Spring GK: Hazards of lithium prophylaxis. *Dis Nerv Syst* 35:351-354, 1974

51. Paykel ES, Mueller PS, De La Vergne P: Amitriptyline, weight gain and carbohydrate craving: a side effect. *Br J Psychiatry* 123:501-507, 1973

52. Pope HG, Hudson JI, Jonas JM, et al: Bulimia treated with imipramine: a placebo-controlled double-blind study. *Am J Psychiatry* 140:554-558, 1983

53. Walsh BT, Stewart JW, Wright L, et al: Treatment of bulimia with monoamine oxidase inhibitors. *Am J Psychiatry* 139:1629-1630, 1982

Afterword

As clinical researchers deeply committed to understanding the interaction between mind and brain for both clinical and theoretical purposes, we would have been delighted to present a practical integration of these chapters. However, we find ourselves unable to grasp the remarkable complexity of chemical and verbal influences on brain function with sufficient clarity to formulate a concluding chapter. We expect to see integrative models in the near future.

Index